Your Miracle in Making

Your Miracle in Making

Explaining the Journey of Motherhood

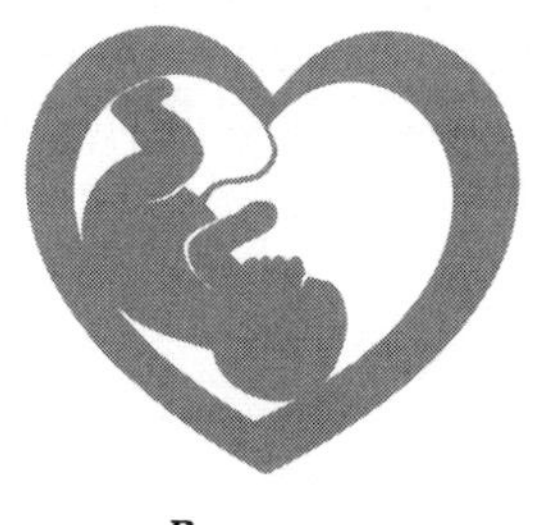

Pregnancy

Dr. Himanshu Bavishi

Bavishi Fertility Institute

Prabhat Paperbacks

Published by
PRABHAT PAPERBACKS
4/19 Asaf Ali Road,
New Delhi-110 002 (INDIA)
e-mail: prabhatbooks@gmail.com

ISBN 978-93-89982-72-5
YOUR MIRACLE IN MAKING
by Dr. Himanshu Bavishi

Edition
First, 2020

Price
₹ 300.00 (Rupees Three Hundred only)

Printed at
R-Tech Offset Printers, Delhi

Preface

"A safe pregnancy and genius child do not just happen" but it is a collective effort of conscious, well informed, actively involved parents and their medical service providers.

In spite of rapid developments, science has not been able to produce life. Bringing a new life to this world is no less than a miracle. When you are bringing a new life to the world, it is very very special for you, your family, your near and dear ones, your society, nation and the world.

Pregnancy is the most enjoyable phase in the life of a woman. Mood, atmosphere and attitude of the whole family change. A lot of preparations are to be done for the new arrival.

Correct scientific information in concise, easy-to-understand and utilisable format empowers pregnant women. Correct and scientific knowledge on physical and emotional changes, common symptoms and remedies, ideal nutrition, child development, proper ante and post-natal care and childbirth are an essential tool and help a would-be-mother to cope with the changes as they evolve in a pregnancy.

This book is a compilation of the latest information of medical science and the wisdom of ancient sciences like 'Garbh Sanskar' with its modern relevance.

Through the inclusion of easy-to-understand terms, accurate medical information, real-life scenarios of conditions that could occur during pregnancy (and how to handle them), this book gives pregnant women the power to maximise their chances of having a successful pregnancy, delivery and, ultimately, a healthy baby.

Bavishi Fertility Institute is a premiere fertility treatment institute of India and the world. We have a vast experience of treating pregnancies, more importantly, high-risk and precious pregnancies. We value the importance of safe journey of pregnancy and childbirth, and have, hence, done the hard work to help maximum couples and families fulfil their dream of a complete family safely and make their journey of parenthood enjoyable and fulfilling.

'Your Miracle in Making', published in four languages—English, Gujarati, Hindi and Marathi, is a book very meticulously prepared for the 'to-be parents'.

This book gives you all the information you need about your pregnancy.

Contents

1
Pregnancy at a Glance

Whenever one thinks of pregnancy, the fact of fertilization is a basic need. Conception is the process that begins with fertilization of an egg with sperm and ends with the implantation of an embryo in the mother's uterus.

Natural Conception

A woman conceives around the time she is ovulating, i.e., when the egg has been released from her one of the ovaries.

During intercourse (sex) sperms are ejaculated from a man's penis into a woman's vagina. In one ejaculation, there may be millions of sperms, but most of the sperms leak out with the semen out of vagina, but some manage to swim up through cervix and reach its destination. In an ovulating woman, cervical fluid facilitates sperm transportation into

Fertilization

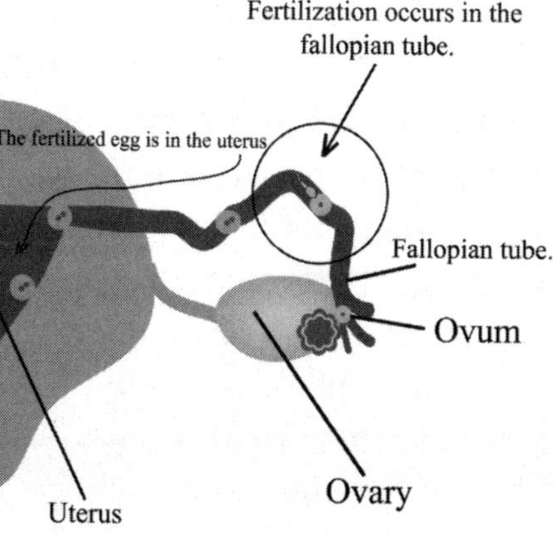

the fallopian tubes. Fertilization actually takes place in the fallopian tube.

Within 4-6 days of fertilization, the embryo (fertilized egg) moves down slowly through the fallopian tube to the uterus and continues growing after getting embedded in it. The embryo attaches itself to the uterus and this is called **implantation**. After implantation, the embryo – the body – begins to produce hormones which support pregnancy. Hormonal release from an embryo prevents the uterus lining (endometrial) from being shed. This is the reason why a woman misses her period when she is pregnant.

During pregnancy, hormone levels change.

This increase in hormone level may cause the following effects:

You may:

- have mood swings.
- feel easily irritable.
- feel nauseous, have a tendency to vomit.
- heaviness in epigastrium (upper abdomen)/ acidity.
- feel uneasiness etc.

But these effects become less prominent, and these disappear or change slowly around 3 months of pregnancy.

Best time to get pregnant

A woman is most likely to get pregnant if she has intercourse (sex) within 24 hours of ovulation. Ovulation usually takes place at around the 14th day of normal, regular 28 days of her menstrual cycle.

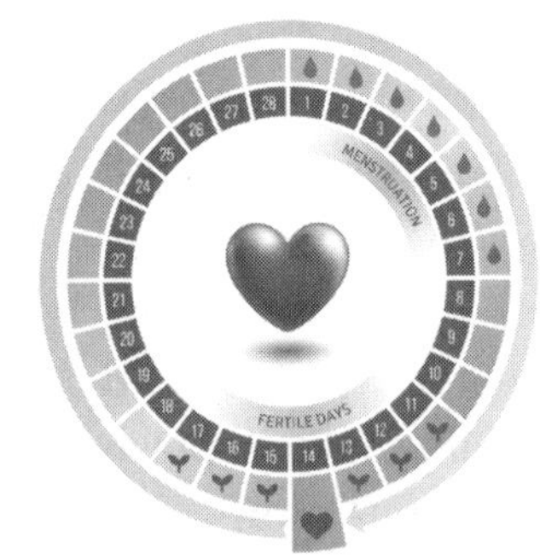

An egg lives for about 12-24 hours after its release, during which it should be fertilized by a sperm. A sperm can live up to 72 hours in a woman's body.

Sperm will decide a boy or a girl

Every cell of the body contains 46 chromosomes (tiny thread like structures carrying about 2,000 genes). Sperm and egg have half the number of chromosomes (23 chromosomes each). After fertilization, the embryo has 46 chromosomes, 23 from father and 23 from mother. The female egg always contains X chromosome, whereas the male sperm can have either X chromosome or Y chromosome. Hence, when the egg and sperm meet, the sperm decides whether the baby will be a boy (XY) or a girl (XX).

A healthy pregnancy keeps everybody happy

Whenever you start thinking about pregnancy or trying for pregnancy, try to be healthy from the start, even before pregnancy and maintain your health before, during and after pregnancy.

Remember that it can take a year to be pregnant. It is a good idea to consult a doctor when you try for a pregnancy for evaluation of your health and optimise your nutrition. If you are trying from one year or more and remain unsuccessful, then it is better to consult your doctor soon to find out the reason for not conceiving.

You may visit your doctor particularly so:

- If your age is more than 30 years.
- You have had any previous illness.
- Any operation in your pelvis.
- Any health issue with your husband, etc.

There are few things to be taken care of to help you stay on healthy side.

- Start changing your dietary habit and schedule. Include more healthy food in your diet. Avoid eating processed, unhealthy and junk food.
- *Exercise:* It is very important to control your weight before getting pregnant as it will help you to stay in shape during pregnancy. Weight reduction can lower your risk of miscarriage and has been proven to help reduce pregnancy and labour complications.
- Educate yourself about pregnancy, body changes during it, stages of pregnancy and labour, delivery/ birth, when you consult a doctor.
- Talk to your doctor or relatives to get knowledge and their experience about pregnancy. Share their experience of parenthood.
- Visit your dentist before you get pregnant for dental check-up. Brush your teeth daily.
- Stop smoking and taking alcohol.
- Ask your hubby to join you on new habit change. Let him know about changes you get, your emotions every time and let him enjoy his fatherhood too.
- Develop a habit of reading books and literature that calms your mind and soul. Avoid watching violent shows and movies. Develop a habit of listening to light music.
- Take rest whenever you can. Even a nap is refreshing.
- Join a class of prenatal yoga or prenatal exercise.
- Avoid chemicals that could possibly harm your body which may be present at your workplace, at your home or anywhere.

- Whenever you visit medical or paramedical person, tell them that you are pregnant. This can prevent exposure to harmful tests and chemicals.
- Daily drink 6 to 8 glasses of water.
- Add 300-500 calories a day while pregnant.
- Know about signs of premature labour and its warning signs to call the doctor.
- Take a breastfeeding class to help and prepare yourself for it.
- Keep your bag ready to go to the birth centre or hospital.

□

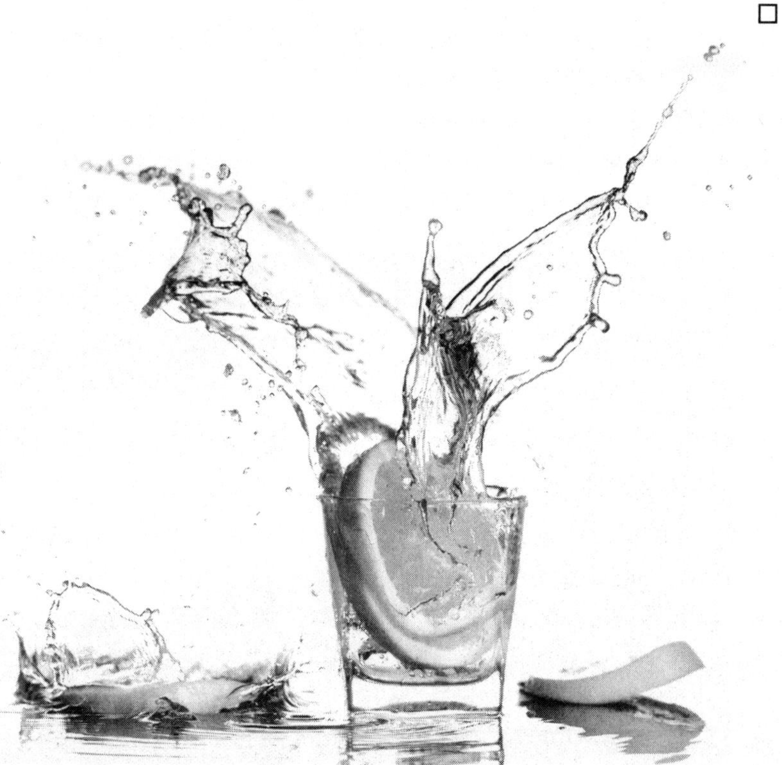

2

Diagnosis of Pregnancy

The beginning of pregnancy may be detected in a number of different ways either by medical testing or without it.

These are some common symptoms that can signify pregnancy:

- Like nausea, vomiting, excessive tiredness, fatigue.
- Craving for certain foods that are normally not considered a favourite food.
- Frequent urination.
- Missed menstrual period.
- There are blood and urine tests that can detect pregnancy, 12 days after implantation.

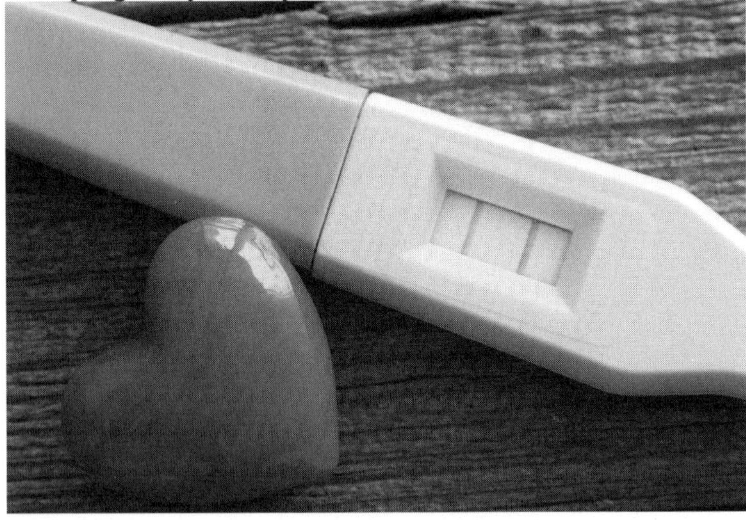

- Blood test is more accurate than urine test.
- Blood test is Serum Beta HCG level. It is most accurate. It may be conducted serially.
- Home pregnancy test is urine test conducted with a test kit that detects changes in the urine composition.

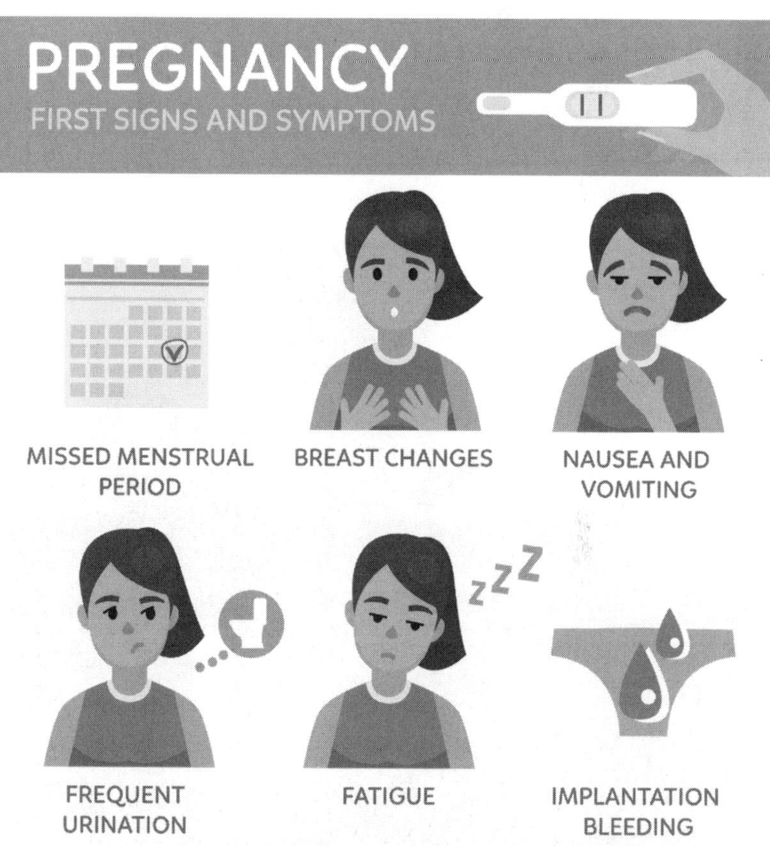

- You can check your morning urine sample in strip. On the device, the appearance of two lines in the result window is an indication of pregnancy.

- Ultrasonography, but it can be useful only after 3-4 weeks of fertilization.
- It can detect small gestational sac as early as 4-5 weeks by transvaginal ultrasound.
- It can detect a gestational sac (a bag of water in which the pregnancy develops) with a yolk sac as early as 5 weeks.
- It can detect embryo as early as 5 weeks and 3 days.
- It can detect foetal heartbeat as early as 6 weeks.

□

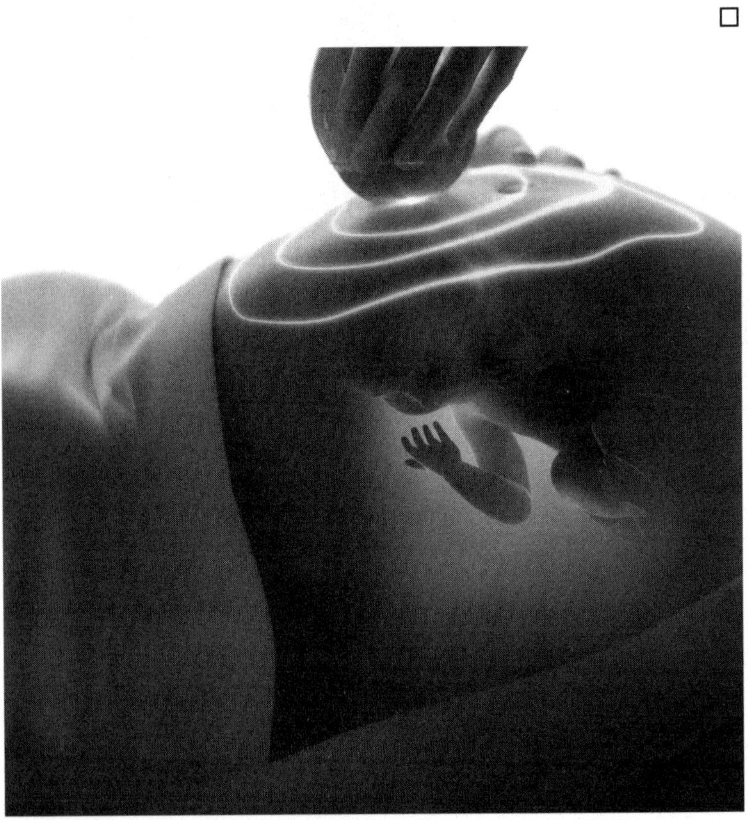

3
Pregnancy Week by Week

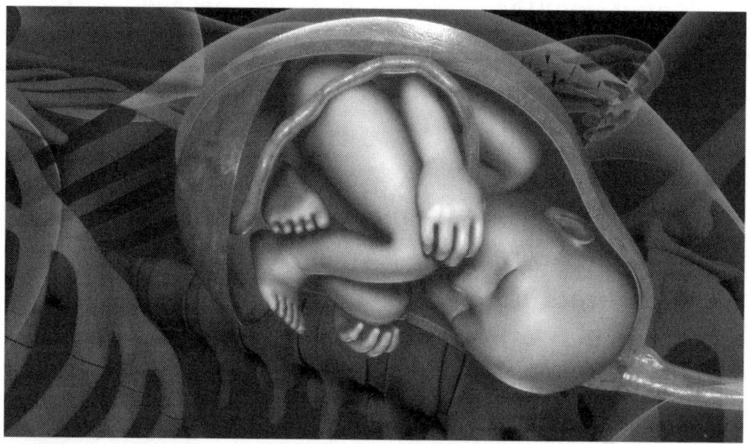

In the previous chapter, you have read about the process of getting pregnant, tips to keep in mind and how to detect and confirm pregnancy.

Now there are a few things on your mind, such as:

- What is your current week/age of pregnancy?
- How may your baby look like in the womb today?
- How much may your baby weigh and measure in length at the present stage of pregnancy?

Some of the common terminologies:

Embryo: From conception to 8th week.

Foetus: From 9th week till birth of baby.

Gestational age (Menstrual age): Starts from 1st day of your LMP (last menstrual period).

Mostly used by doctors.

Average gestational age at delivery is 40 weeks.

Ovulatory age (Fertilization age): Starts from the day you conceive. Average ovulatory age at delivery is 38 weeks.

Trimester: There are 3 trimesters in human pregnancy. Each trimester consists of 13 weeks.

Lunar months: A pregnancy lasts an average of 10 lunar months (28 days each), hence, 280 days in total.

Due date calculation: Your doctor will always calculate your due date from the 1st day of your LMP. For instance, 9 months +7 days in your 1st day of LMP.

The average length and weight of baby varies from baby to baby and from one pregnancy to other.

Umbilical cord: The umbilical cord is a baby's lifeline. It is the link between you and your baby. Blood circulates through the cord, carrying oxygen and food to the baby and carrying waste away.

Placenta: The placenta is attached to the lining of the uterus and separates your baby's circulation from your circulation. In the placenta, oxygen and food from your bloodstream pass into your baby's bloodstream and are carried to your baby along, the umbilical cord. Antibodies that give resistance to infection pass to your baby in the same way. Alcohol, nicotine and other drugs can also pass to your baby this way.

Amniotic sac: Inside the uterus, the baby floats in a bag of fluid called the amniotic sac. Before or during labour, the sac or 'membrane' breaks and the fluid drains out. This is known as the 'water breaking'.

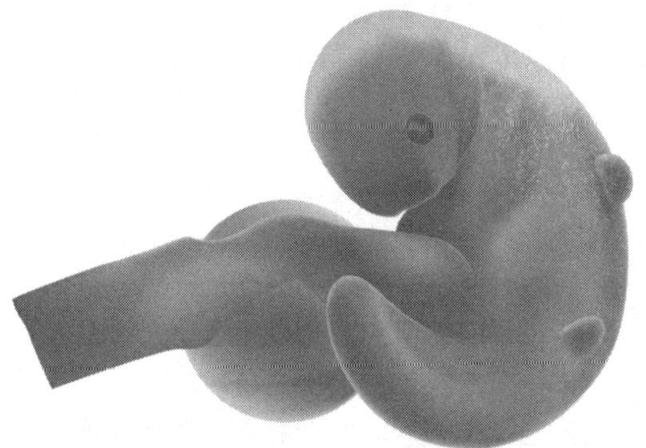

Heart beat run between 80 and 150 times per minute and internal organs begin forming

6 Weeks' Pregnancy

Changes in foetus:

- From crown (top of the head) to rump (bottom of buttocks), your baby measures 2-4 mm or 0.08-0.16 inch, the size of a small lentil.
- Heart is the size of poppy seed and beating on its own.
- Your baby has its own bloodstream with blood circulating already.
- Within 5 months, more than 100s of billions of neurons are formed in the brain.
- Embryos are 10,000 times larger than the egg.

Changes in you:

- You may lose some weight because of not eating well and nausea.
- Abdominal changes are not apparent.
- The areolas darken to brownish circle of patches around the nipples.

- Bluish vein may be seen under the skin of breasts.
- You may be prone to fatigue and nausea.

7 Weeks' Pregnancy

Changes in foetus:

- From crown to rump, your baby measures 4-5 mm or 0.16-0.20 inches, the size of a small raspberry.
- Beating heart is observed.
- Baby's intestine, heart chambers and brain hemisphere are formed.
- Eyes and nostrils are formed.
- Small protruding buds are also seen that develop in ears and limbs.
- The skull is still transparent and the brain is growing fast.

Changes in you:

- Weight gain is still less.
- In many patients, it may be lost due to nausea, vomiting and inadequate intake of food.

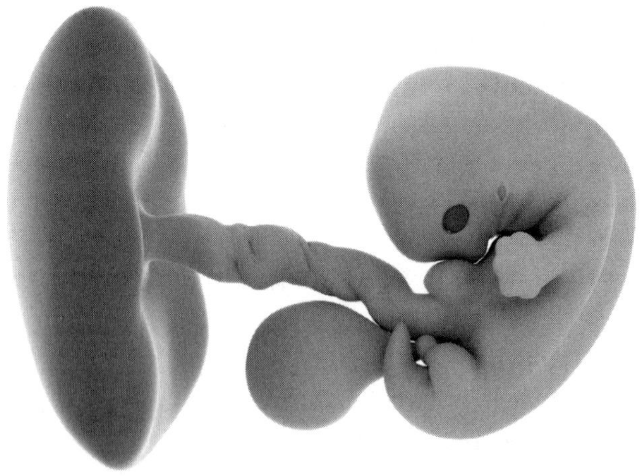

- You may have symptoms like nausea, vomiting, fatigue, indigestion, constipation, etc.
- Mucus plug (sticky discharge) is also established in cervix and it may come out from the vagina. If it is not associated with itching or foul smell, then it is normal (physiological).
- You may have dreams and fantasies about your baby and these are the true beginnings of your emotional bonding.

8 Weeks' Pregnancy

Changes in foetus:

- From crown to rump, your baby measures 14-20 mm or 0.50-0.75 inches, size of pinto bean. (type of Rajma)
- Now your baby graduates from an embryo to a foetus.
- All main internal organs are present.
- Baby has recognisable human face with nostrils, lips and mouth with tongue.
- This baby is covered with skin but is still translucent.
- Baby has started moving inside the uterus, but you will not be able to feel it.
- Toes and fingers begin to form. Paddle-shaped feet and hands are present.
- Baby's eyelid begins to form and until it completes, the eye will appear open.
- Digestive tract is growing continuously.
- Ten dental buds form in each jaw.
- Heart function is fully developed with pumping approximately 150 beats per minute.
- Umbilical cord is clearly visible.

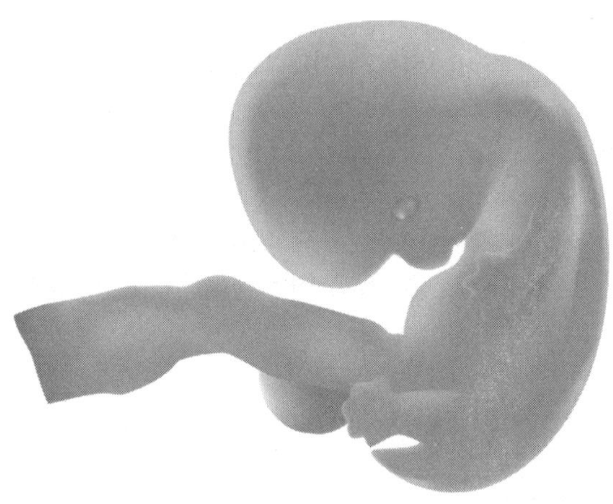

The brain cells are developing. Eyes and ears are becoming noticeable, hands and feet are emerging from developing arms and legs

Changes in you:

- Uterus is of the size of a tennis ball.
- Because of hormonal changes, you may have mood swings similar to premenstrual tension.
- Your metabolic rate is increasing 10-25%.
- Your uterus tightens, contracts and relaxes throughout pregnancy, but you may not feel it.
- You may have constipation.
- You may have insomnia, nausea, vomiting.

9 Weeks' Pregnancy

Changes in foetus:

- From crown to rump, your baby measures 22-30 mm or 1-1.25 inches, of the size of green olive.
- Baby looks like tadpole and more human.

- Hands and feet continue to grow along the fingers, toes and elbows.
- Internal organs, such as ovaries, testes, pancreas, intestine, gallbladder and anus have formed, but we cannot make out external genitalia.

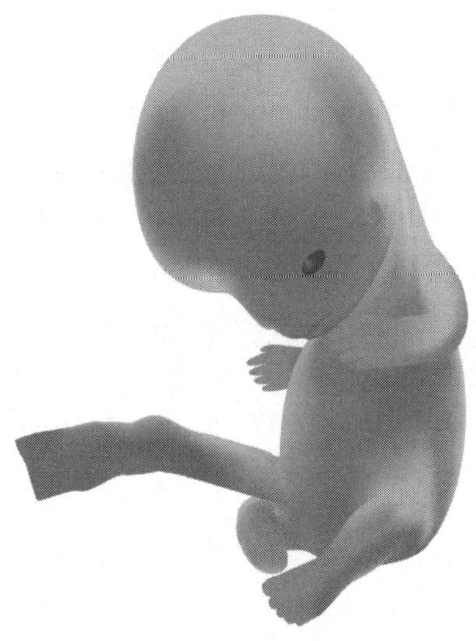

Critical portion development is nearly finished. Baby's head is about half his length, Facial features are quite recognisable

Changes in you:

- Your waistline may start to thicken.
- Your HCG level is at peak in this week.
- Your first trimester's symptoms may continue.
- Your belly's shape may be changed. You may have increased vaginal discharge that is normal in pregnancy.
- You may have a metallic taste in your mouth.

10 Weeks' Pregnancy

Changes in foetus:

- From crown to rump, your baby measures 31-42 mm or 1.25-1.75 inches.
- Baby has started to put on weight. Your baby's weight is approximately 5 gm or 0.18 oz.
- Prenatal test CVS (Chorionic Villus Sampling) usually conducted from this week to 12th week.
- You can come to know about many congenital malformations that occur during embryonic period.
- All vital organs have formed.
- Tail has disappeared totally.
- Finger and toes are no longer webbed.
- Skeleton, bones are starting to form.
- Rapid brain development is taking place with almost 2,50,000 neurons being produced every minute.

Changes in you:

- You may or may not gain few kgs of weight by now, but you may lose weight due to nausea and vomiting.
- Abdominal changes are still not apparent.
- You may have spotting or brownish discharge that is called implantation bleeding. If excessive, consult your doctor.
- You may have tender breast, mild cramps in lower abdomen.

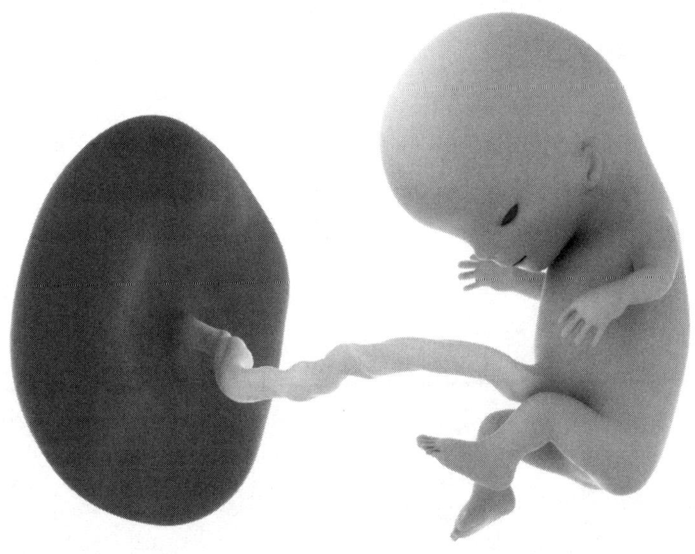

11 Weeks' Pregnancy

Changes in foetus:

- From crown to rump, your baby measures 44-60 mm or 1.50-2.50 inches, of the size of peanut.
- Foetus weight is 8 gm or 0.3 oz.
- Baby increases 30-fold and triple in length.
- Blood vessels in placenta are multiplying to keep up with nutrient supply to foetus.
- External genital shows obvious differences but it would be more complete after 13 weeks.
- Baby can open its mouth and close its fist, and can suck thumb. Heartbeat is 120-160/BPM (beats per minute).

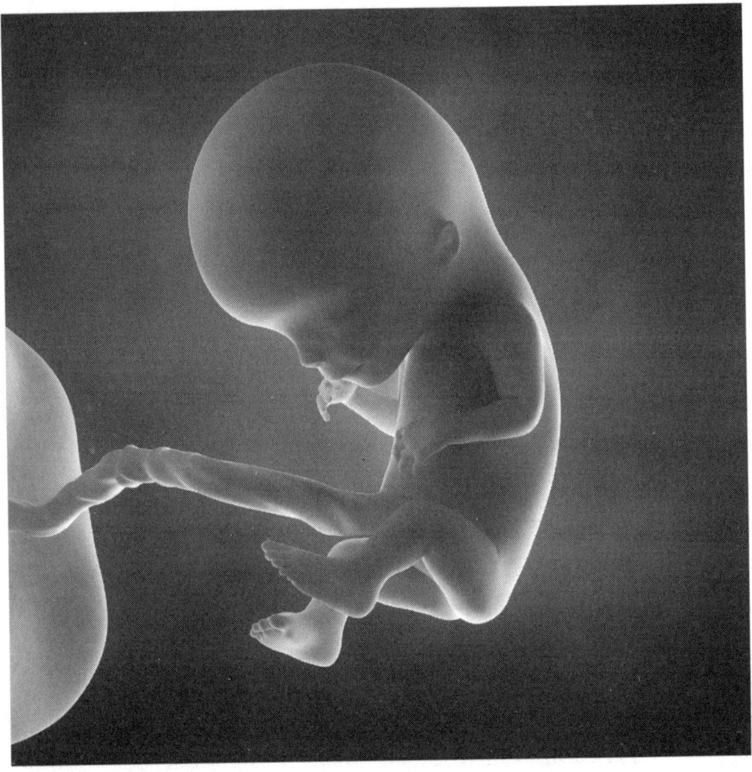

Changes in you:

- Some women experience glowing skin while others suffer from acne.
- Some feel changes like hair and nail growth and hair loss.
- You have leg cramps that are most common, but it is not harmful. It is due to mineral and vitamin deficiency or it may be due to your leg not being able to tolerate the weight of a pregnant uterus.
- You may have mood swings also.

12 Weeks' Pregnancy

Changes in foetus:

- From crown to rump, your baby measures 60 mm or 2.50 inches, size of plum.
- Foetus weight is 14 gm or 0.5 oz.
- It is the end of the first trimester.
- Baby is active, moving in the uterus.
- Baby is swallowing amniotic fluid, can pass urine which constitutes the amniotic fluid.
- Baby has wrist, ankles, elbows, fingers and toes with nails and can make a fist.
- Baby's head is quite large in proportion to body.
- Baby is floating in amniotic fluid that is approximately 100 ml.

Changes in you:

- Your risk of miscarriage drops significantly.
- You may develop black line (dark) on your abdomen called the linea nigra which will fade after birth.
- You may gain 10% of total pregnancy weight or you may lose also.
- You may have frequency of urination and bleeding gums due to hormonal changes.
- Now your uterus will grow up just about the pelvic cavity, so you may have less pressure on your bladder.
- Your breast size increases.

13 Weeks' Pregnancy

Changes in foetus:

- From crown to rump, your baby measures 65-78 mm or 3 inches.
- Foetus weight is 20 gm or 1 oz.
- Baby's vocal cord forms.
- Baby is hiccuping now. So, this will strengthen the diaphragm and prepare the respiratory system for breathing.
- Kidneys makes urine and bone marrow makes white blood cells for fighting against infection after birth.
- All the baby's organs, nerves and muscles are formed and now start functioning together.
- Baby's eyelids are fused together and will not reopen till 30 weeks to protect the developing eyes.

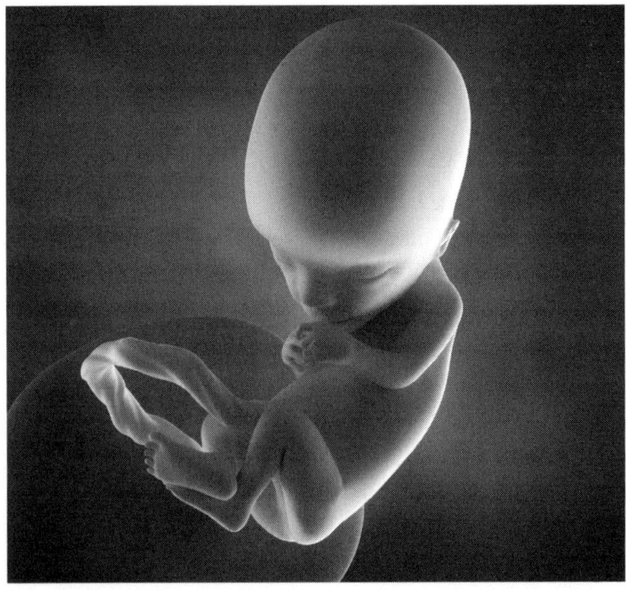

Changes in you:

- You will feel better and less sick.
- Your shoes will beginning to feel tight.
- You may have chances of getting urinary tract infection very frequently. So, ensure good liquid intake.

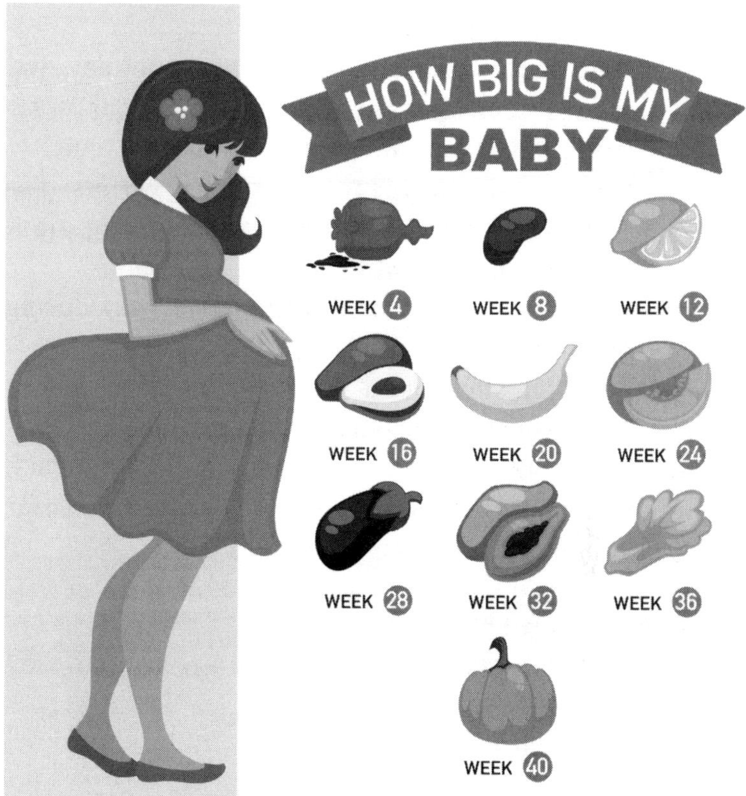

What to keep in mind during pregnancy

As your baby is totally dependent on you for all its needs, you should eat properly, rest enough and stay as healthy as possible throughout the phase of pregnancy.

About food

1. Avoid fatty and greasy food, carbonated drinks, junk food and processed meals.
2. Eat slowly.
3. Take healthy, balanced diet and fresh food.
4. Take plenty of water, juices and food rich in fibre to avoid constipation.
5. Take frequent small meals, 5-6 times per day, that relaxes your stomach and maintains your sugar level rather than eating one full meal at a time.
6. You may take all types of fruits and dry fruits.
7. Take high protein diet like sprouted moong, black gram, rajma and chikki, etc.
8. You need an additional 300 calories/day during pregnancy.
9. Avoid junk food or outside food.
10. Take biscuits or bhakhari in the morning.
11. If you still feel nauseous and vomiting tendency, you can try a remedy – soak cucumber in water for 10 minutes and then eat it.

About habits and hygiene

1. Avoid lying flat on your back, try propping yourself to avoid heartburn.
2. Try to sleep in lateral positions.
3. Remain stress-free.
4. You can do yoga, walking, swimming, etc. if you don't have any problem.
5. You can listen to soft soothing music or read inspiring books.

6. If you want to do hair dye/hair colour, you can do it, but you may not get proper result because of hormonal changes. It is not harmful to foetus.
7. Avoid smoking, tobacco chewing throughout pregnancy.
8. Maintain strict standards of hygiene and cleanliness and wash your hands with soap each and every time before you eat.
9. Restrict tea and coffee intake.

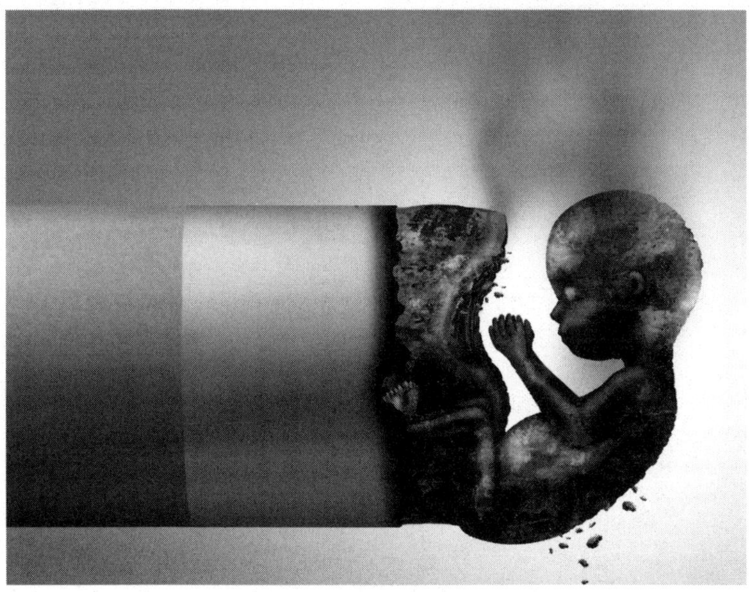

10. Avoid polluted air.
11. You may feel the size of your clothes have changed gradually.
12. Don't wear too tight clothing.

PREGNANT WOMEN
INFOGRAPHIC
RELAX MUSIC MOM & BABY
SOFT SOOTHING MUSIC WILL RELAX YOU AND THE BABY
POSITIONS FOR SLEEPING
AVOID LYING FLAT ON YOUR BACK
TRY PROPPING YOURSELF TO AVOID HEARTBURN.
TRY TO SLEEP IN LATERAL POSITIONS
HEALTH CHECK
VISIT YOUR DOCTOR FOR REGULAR CHECK UPS AND FOLLOW HIS ADVICE
RED BLOOD CELL PRODUCTION
STEM CELL PRODUCTION
BONES AND TEETH HEALTHY
YOGA
AVOID STRSS AND DO YOGA REGULARLY
HEALTHY FOOD
CARBOHYDRATE
IRON
CALCIUM
VITAMIN
PROTEIN
FOOD TO AVOID
SPICY
COFFEE
CANNED FOOD
BEER AND ALCOHOL
SALT
MSG
VERY SALTY
MONOSODIUM GLUTAMATE
CONSULTATION WITH DOCTOR
NO SMOKING

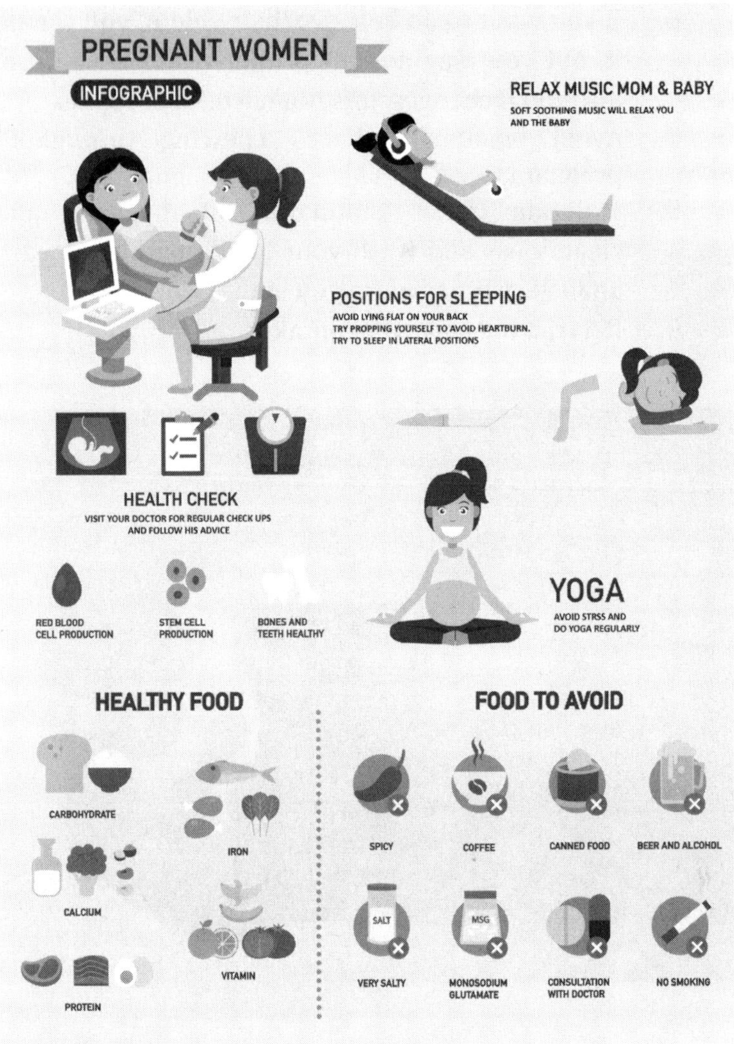

13. Your entire blood circulation system increases during pregnancy. So, you may feel dizziness, dehydration, headache, sweaty and flushed feeling.
14. You have to visit doctor regularly.

15. If you have swelling on your legs, contact your doctor and keep your legs elevated.
16. If you have pain in abdomen or a watery discharge consult your doctor.
17. You should check for checklist of hospitalisation.

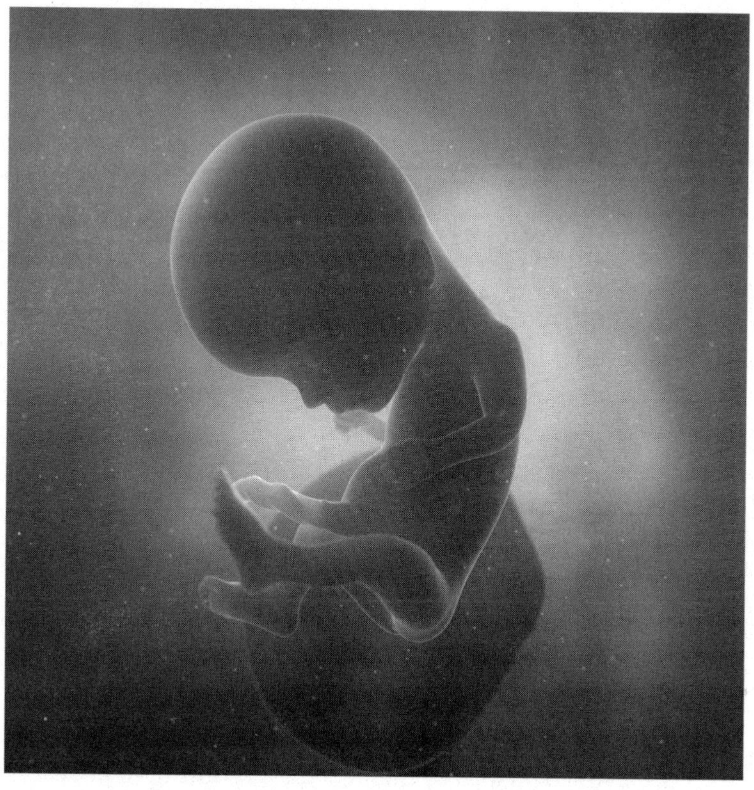

14 Weeks' Pregnancy

Changes in foetus:

- From crown to rump, your baby measures 78-85 mm or 3-4 inches.

- Foetus weight is approximately 20 gm or 1 oz.
- Reproductive organs of the baby are developed.
- Thyroid gland begins its function.
- Baby's skin is very thin, head hair and eyebrows are growing.
- Bone marrow has begun to produce blood cells which were previously produced by yolk sac.
- Now your baby is yawning, stretching or wiggling her toes and fingers, but you cannot feel all these movements.

Changes in you:

- Some women begin producing colostrum or pre-milk.
- Your all first trimester symptoms may end-up or you feel better than earlier.
- You can feel your uterus just above the pelvic region.

15-22 Weeks' Pregnancy

Changes in foetus:

- Baby is growing faster than any other time in their life.
- Head and body are more in proportion.
- The face becomes much more defined and nails, eyebrows and eyelashes are beginning to grow.
- Your baby has its own fingerprint, footprint. The fingernails and toenails are growing and hands can grip.
- At 22 weeks' your baby is covered in very fine soft hair called lanugo.

- Muscle tissue and bone continue to form, creating a more complete skeleton.
- Skin begins to form.
- Meconium develops in your baby's intestinal tract. It is the first bowel movement.
- Sucking motion with mouth is developing.
- The baby is more active and you may feel a fluttering feeling in your abdomen.
- Baby is covered by fine, hairy lanugo and a greasy substance called vernix. This protects the skin.
- Eyebrows, eyelashes, fingernails and toenails, have formed. Your baby can scratch itself.
- Baby can hear and swallow.
- Size approximately 10-11 cm (at 15 weeks) to 27-30 cm (at 22 weeks), weight approximately 100 (at 15 weeks) 500 (22 weeks) gm.

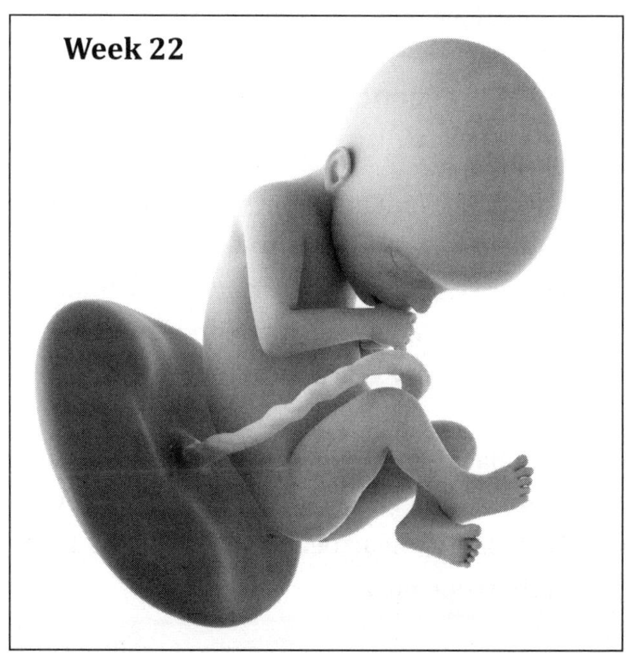

Changes in you:

- You may have gained weight approximately up to 4 kg.
- You can feel your baby's movement for the first time after 20-22 weeks and if it is your second pregnancy, you will feel earlier approximately at 16-18 weeks.
- Your first trimester symptoms have almost gone away except that you can have occasional nausea due to acidity.
- At first, you may feel fluttering/bubbling or slight shifting movement.
- Sometimes you will see a bump that is clearly hand/foot.
- Now the height of your uterus has grown to just below the navel.

23-30 Weeks' Pregnancy

Changes in foetus:

- Baby is now moving about vigorously and responds to touch and sound.
- Baby is swallowing small amount of amniotic fluid and is passing urine in amniotic fluid.
- Your baby may get hiccups and you can feel it by a jerk.
- Your baby also follows a pattern of waking and sleeping. And it may be different from you.
- Your baby's heartbeat can be heard through a stethoscope now.

- Your baby may also be covered by vernix, a greasy substance that disappears after birth.
- From 26 weeks, your baby has a chance of survival if it is born.
- Bone marrow begins to make blood cells.
- Taste buds form on your baby's tongue.
- Real hair begins to grow on your baby's head.
- Lungs are formed but not working.
- Baby's reproductive organs begin to set their proper place.
- At 26 weeks, your baby's eyelids open for the first time.
- Your baby is of the size of 11 to 17 inch in length and weight is up to approximately 500 gms at 23 weeks to 1.7 kg at 30 weeks.

Changes in you:

- You have gained weight and it is approximately 1 kg per month.
- The height of your uterus grows to just above the level of your navel.
- You feel a lot of movement of Foetus at this time.
- You may have acidity problem as uterus is growing.
- You have swelling in legs and hands. It is common in pregnancy, but you have to check your blood pressure regularly.
- You may have stretch marks on your tummy or thighs. Your breast size has increased.

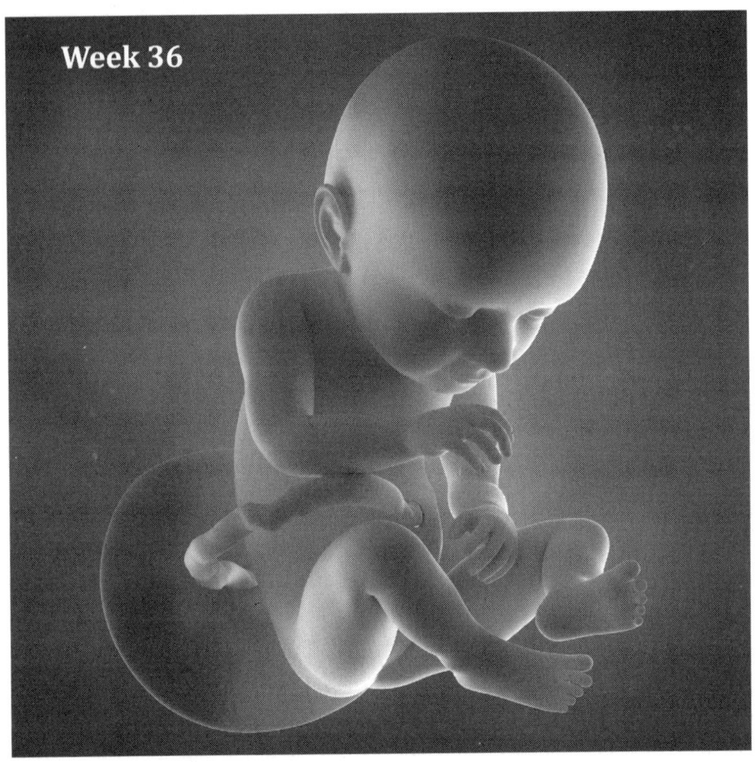

31-36 Weeks' Pregnancy

Changes in foetus:

- Baby is continuously growing.
- Skin becomes smooth and lanugo disappears, but vernix gets thickened.
- Regular talking, reading and singing to yourself while you are pregnant will help you bond with your baby before birth.
- Baby gains weight by half pound/week.
- Bones are fully formed but soft.
- Baby's kicks are very forceful.

- As baby is growing very fast, baby has less space to move around. So you can feel only stretching and wiggles like movement at the end of 35 weeks.
- Now baby can open and close eyes and sense changes in light.
- Lungs are not fully formed but breathing movement occurs.
- Baby's body begins to store minerals and vitamins.
- Your baby measures 16-19 inches in length and weight approximately 1.5 kg to 2.6 kg.

Changes in you:

- The height of uterus reaches up to chest just below the ribs.
- You have discomfort in breathing, pain around lower ribs, swelling in legs and hands.
- Sometimes you may develop stretch marks on your abdomen and thighs.
- You may have itching on your abdomen due to stretching of skin.
- You can feel tightening and relaxation of your uterus.
- You have to go frequently for urination.

37-40 Weeks' Pregnancy

Changes in foetus:

- From crown to rump, your baby measures approximately 19-21 inches and weights approximately 2.8 kg to 3.5 kg.
- Baby is now considered full term.
- Baby's organs are ready to function on their own.

- Your baby may turn into head-down position for birth.

Changes in you:

- Swelling in the legs may increase.
- Frequency of urine will also increase as your baby's head is engaged in pelvic cavity.
- You may feel contraction and relaxation of uterus.
- You may have back pain.

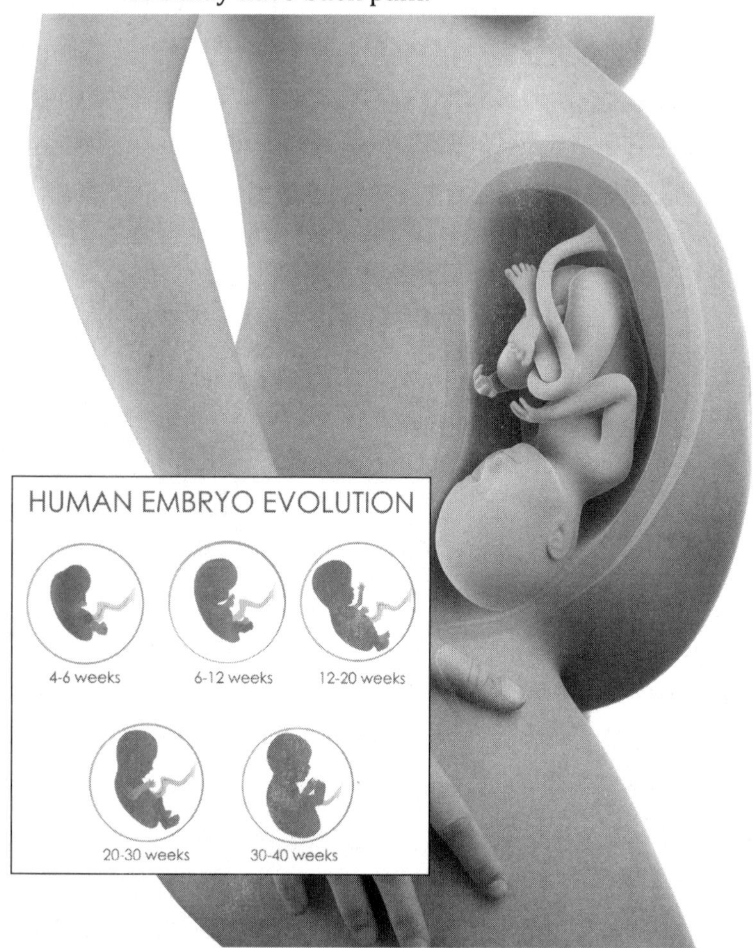

Height and weight chart of fetus

Gestational age	Length (US)	Weight (US)	Length (cm)	Mass (g)
	(crown to rump)		**(crown to rump)**	
8 weeks	0.63 inch	0.04 ounce	1.6 cm	1 gram
9 weeks	0.90 inch	0.07 ounce	2.3 cm	2 grams
10 weeks	1.22 inch	0.14 ounce	3.1 cm	4 grams
11 weeks	1.61 inch	0.25 ounce	4.1 cm	7 grams
12 weeks	2.13 inches	0.49 ounce	5.4 cm	14 grams
13 weeks	2.91 inches	0.81 ounce	7.4 cm	23 grams
14 weeks	3.42 inches	1.52 ounce	8.7 cm	43 grams
15 weeks	3.98 inches	2.47 ounces	10.1 cm	70 grams
16 weeks	4.57 inches	3.53 ounces	11.6 cm	100 grams
17 weeks	5.12 inches	4.94 ounces	13 cm	140 grams
18 weeks	5.59 inches	6.70 ounces	14.2 cm	190 grams
19 weeks	6.02 inches	8.47 ounces	15.3 cm	240 grams
20 weeks	6.46 inches	10.58 ounces	16.4 cm	300 grams
	(crown to heel)		**(crown to heel)**	
20 weeks	10.08 inches	10.58 ounces	25.6 cm	300 grams
21 weeks	10.51 inches	12.70 ounces	26.7 cm	360 grams
22 weeks	10.94 inches	15.17 ounces	27.8 cm	430 grams
23 weeks	11.38 inches	1.10 pound	28.9 cm	501 grams
24 weeks	11.81 inches	1.32 pound	30 cm	600 grams
25 weeks	13.62 inches	1.46 pound	34.6 cm	660 grams
26 weeks	14.02 inches	1.68 pound	35.6 cm	760 grams
27 weeks	14.41 inches	1.93 pound	36.6 cm	875 grams
28 weeks	14.80 inches	2.22 pounds	37.6 cm	1005 grams
29 weeks	15.2 inches	2.54 pounds	38.6 cm	1153 grams
30 weeks	15.71 inches	2.91 pounds	39.9 cm	1319 grams
31 weeks	16.18 inches	3.31 pounds	41.1 cm	1502 grams
32 weeks	16.69 inches	3.75 pounds	42.4 cm	1702 grams
33 weeks	17.20 inches	4.23 pounds	43.7 cm	1918 grams
34 weeks	17.72 inches	4.73 pounds	45 cm	2146 grams
35 weeks	18.19 inches	5.25 pounds	46.2 cm	2383 grams
36 weeks	18.66 inches	5.78 pounds	47.4 cm	2622 grams
37 weeks	19.13 inches	6.30 pounds	48.6 cm	2859 grams
38 weeks	19.61 inches	6.80 pounds	49.8 cm	3083 grams
39 weeks	19.96 inches	7.25 pounds	50.7 cm	3288 grams
40 weeks	20.16 inches	7.63 pounds	51.2 cm	3462 grams
41 weeks	20.35 inches	7.93 pounds	51.7 cm	3597 grams
42 weeks	20.28 inches	8.12 pounds	51.5 cm	3685 grams

The growth of the fetus and the percentile of the ultrasound sonogram during pregnancy is dependent on many factors such as genetic, placental and maternal factors.

Weeks	10th%tile	Average	90th%tile
20	275	412	772
	314	433	790
22	376	496	826
	440	582	882
24	498	674	977
	558	779	1138
26	625	899	1362
	702	1035	1635
28	798	1196	1977
	925	1394	2361
30	1085	1637	2710
	1278	1918	2986
32	1495	2203	3200
	1725	2458	3370
34	1950	2667	3502
	2159	2831	3596
36	2354	2974	3668
	2541	3117	3755
38	2714	3263	3867
	2852	3400	3980
40	2929	3495	4060
	2948	3527	4094
42	2935	3522	1098
	2907	3505	4096
44	2885	3491	4096

□

4

Food and Nutrition in Pregnancy

Nutrition and pregnancy refers to nutritional intake and dietary planning before, during and after pregnancy.

The expecting mom should be very calm and peaceful, and focussed on what they should do for a healthy pregnancy. Eating healthy during pregnancy will help your baby develop and grow and will help to keep you fit and well. You don't need to go on a special diet, but make sure that you eat a variety of foods everyday in order to get right balance of nutrients that you and your baby need.

You might feel more hungry than normal but you do not need to 'eat for two' even if expecting twins or triplets.

Good Routine Food for Vegetarians

What should be included in your daily food to ensure it is a balanced diet?

1. Fruits and vegetables

These provide vitamins, minerals and fibres which help in digestion and prevent constipation. Eat at least five portions of fresh,

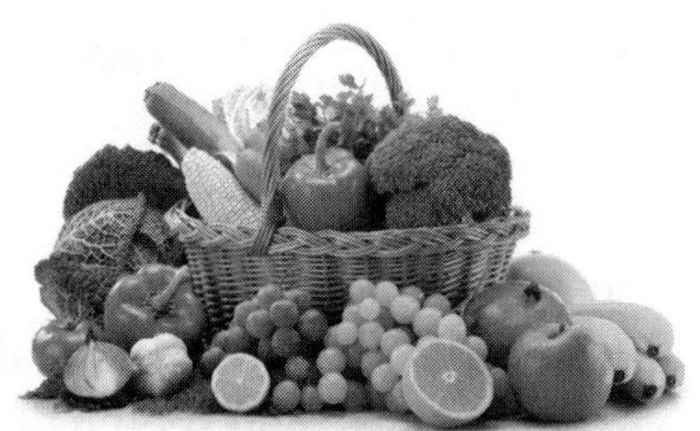

frozen, dried or juicy fruits and vegetables each day, after washing them carefully. Better to eat raw or lightly cooked vegetables.

2. Foods and beverages which are rich in fat

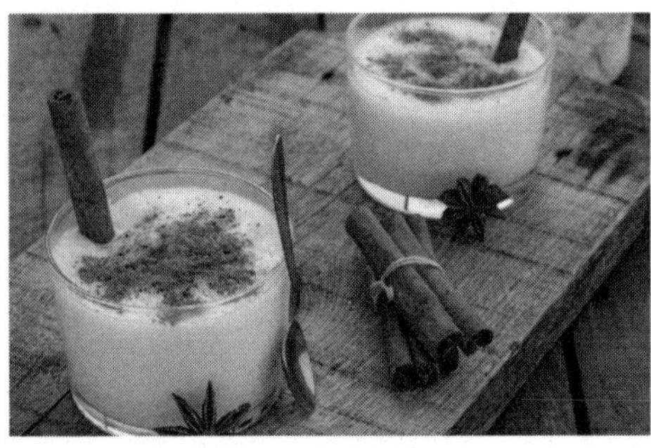

This group includes all oils, ghee, salad dressings, cream, chocolates, biscuits, cake, puddings and sugar-containing drinks. You should eat only a small amount of these foods as sugar contains only calories without providing nutrition to the body. Frequent consumption of such food may cause tooth decay and weight gain. Try to reduce or avoid food that is high in saturated fat and have foods rich in unsaturated fat.

3. Rice, potatoes, bread and other starchy foods

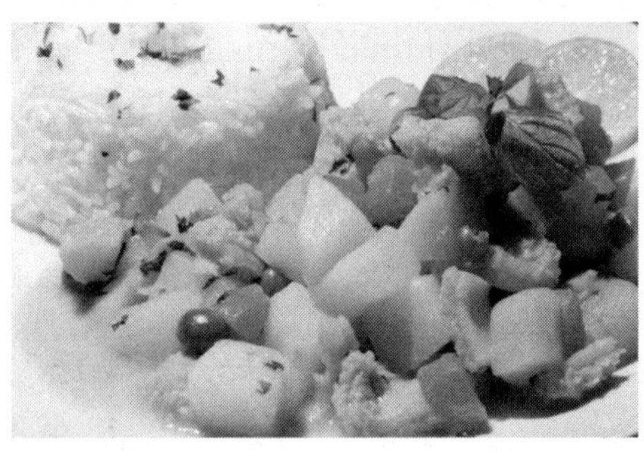

These food types contain carbohydrate which is fit for consumption without containing too much calories. These are also important sources of vitamins and fibres. Such other foods are oats, maize, millet, sweet potatoes, pastas, etc. Such food should be main part of every meal.

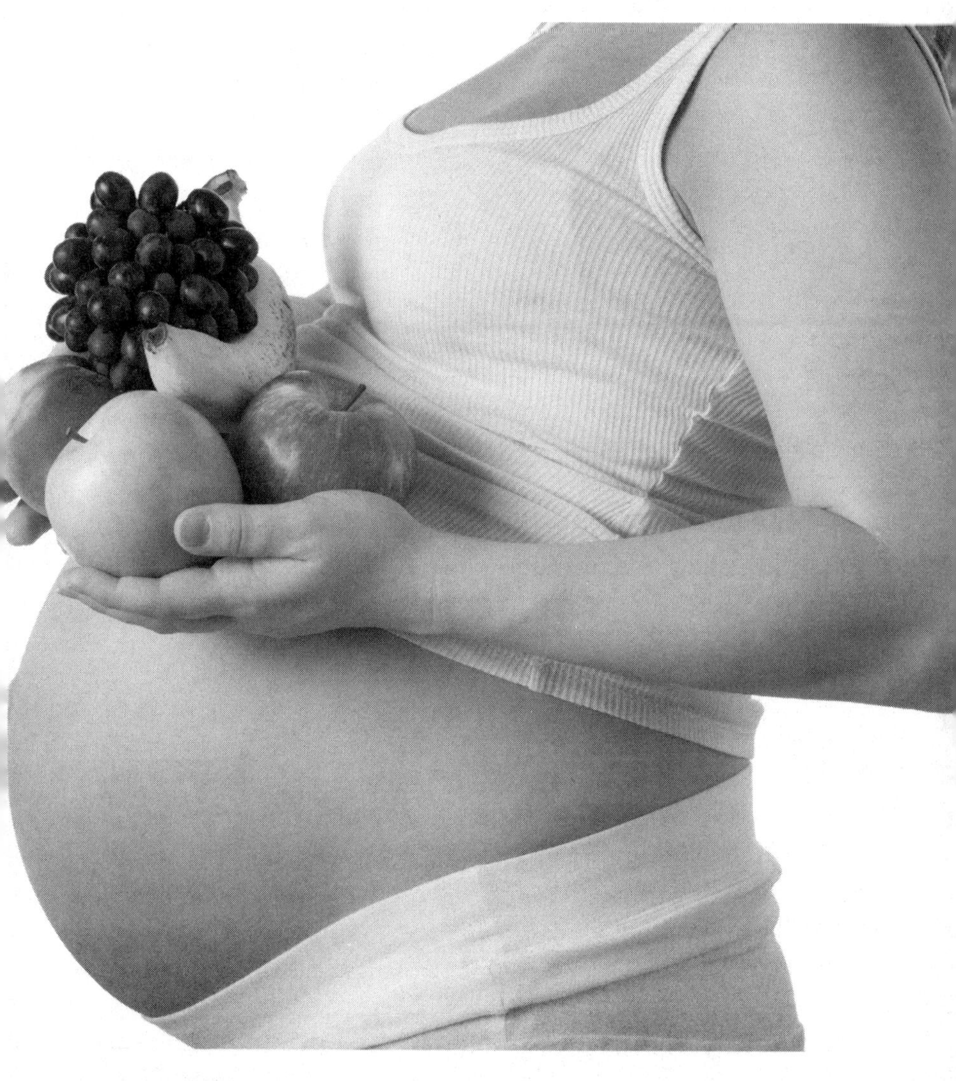

4. High protein diet

For this, you can take Sprouted *Mung*, *Chana* (Black Gram), *Moth*, *Rajma* at least one bowl per day.

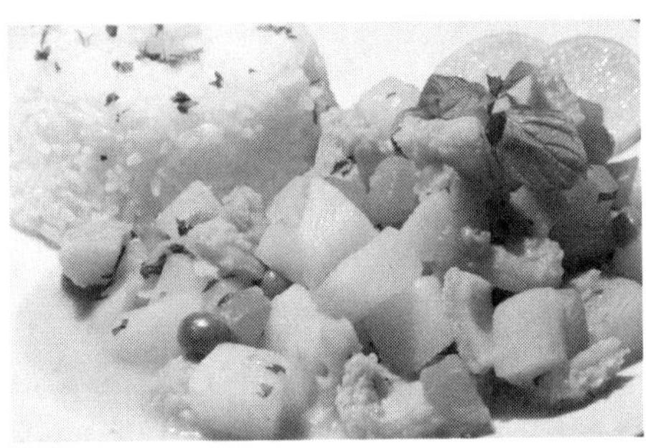

You can take any kind of chikkies like groundnut (shing) chikkies, dry fruit chikkies, dalia's chikkies, etc., preferably made from jaggery rather than sugar.

These foods are main sources of protein. One should eat a moderate amount each day.

5. Milk and dairy products

Milk and its products, like buttermilk, paneer and yoghurt are important. They contain calcium and other nutrients needed by a baby.

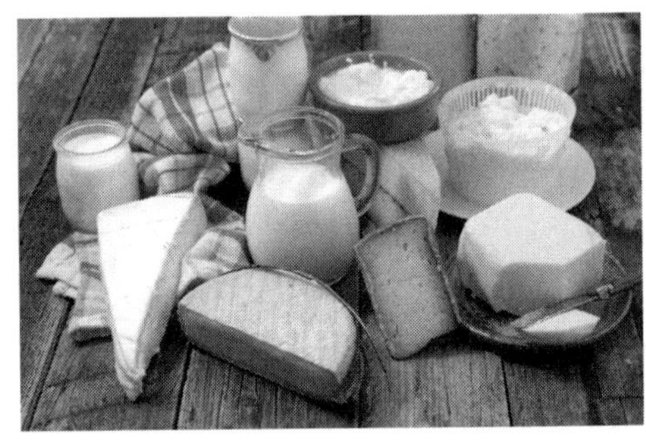

Whenever you take milk, remove the cream from it or use skimmed or low fat-variety milk. You can use low-fat paneer, yoghurt.

6. Healthy drinks and snacks during pregnancy

In addition to other food and fluids, drink 8 to 10 large glasses (at least 2-3 litres) of water a day. A refreshing

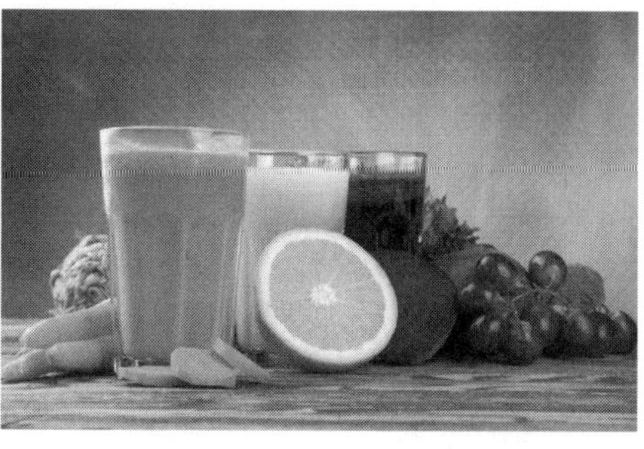

alternative is a glass of chilled filtered water with a twist of lime or mint. There are some other healthy drinks that can be tried, i.e., coconut water, lime juice, skimmed milk and banana shake.

It is best to prepare milk shakes and juices at home and drink them immediately. This reduces risk of any spoilage or contamination. Also be careful while buying drinks from roadside vendors as it is difficult to judge their hygiene and freshness.

There are some tasty and healthy snacks that you would like to take during pregnancy, i.e., grilled paneer tikka (low-fat paneer), fruit and vegetable *bhelpuri*, *dhokla* or *khandvi*, sweet potato chat, steamed or sautéd corn or corn chat, *upma*, mixed vegetable *idli*, *batata poha*, *khakhara*, *shing-chana*, *sev- mamra*, popcorn, etc.

Try to limit or decrease intake of deeply fried or more *ghee*, butter-rich snacks. It is better to use plant oils, rather than animal fat, that are high in saturated fat. Be guided by your appetite, but beware of emotional eating that could make you overeat at times.

Important Elements

1. Requirement of folic acid during pregnancy

It is recommended to take daily a folic acid supplement of 400 mcg before pregnancy (prenatally) and for at least first 12 weeks of pregnancy. It is required to protect your unborn baby against developing neural tube defects, such as *spina bifida*.

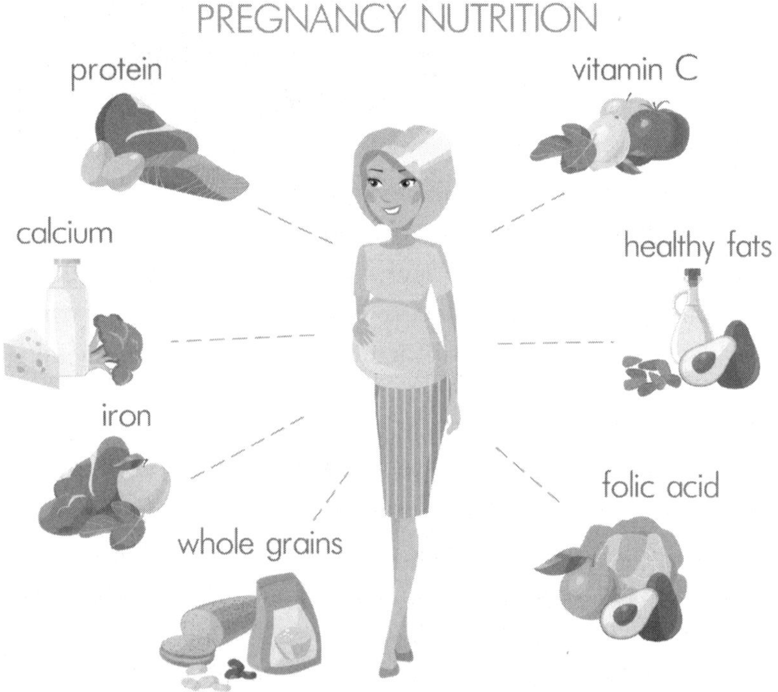

Following are some good sources of folic acid (foliate):

- Green-leafy vegetables like spinach (*palak*), fenugreek leaves (*methi*), corianders (green *dhania*), radish (*muli*), mustard greens, mint (*pudina*), lettuce, etc.
- Pulses like Bengal gram (*chana*), soyabeans, chick peas (*vatana*), kidney beans (*rajma*), etc.

- Vegetables like beetroot, peas, cabbage, French beans (*fansi*), lady's finger (*bhindi*), bottle guard (*dudhi*), carrot (*gaajar*), corn (*makai*) etc.
- Fruits like pomegranate (*anaar*), guava (*amrood*), oranges, sweet lime (*mosambi*), strawberry etc.
- Dry fruits and nuts, like almonds, peanuts (*moongfali*), walnuts, etc.

2. Other vitamins and minerals

A. Vitamin D

Vitamin D is needed to keep bones healthy and to provide baby enough of vitamin D. Vitamin D regulates the amount of calcium and phosphate in the body which keep bones and teeth healthy. Many vegetarian mothers may have deficiency of vitamin D. The best source of vitamin D is sunlight. The time of exposure to sunlight to get vitamin D is different for different persons as it depends on skin type, time of the day and a year.

B. Iron

Deficiency of iron leads to anaemia (low haemoglobin) which causes weakness and fatigue. Food rich in iron includes green-leafy vegetables, jaggery, beetroot, carrots, millets, dry fruits (figs, black raisins) dates, etc. It is also supplied in the form of tablets and syrups throughout pregnancy by a doctor.

C. Vitamin C

It helps to absorb iron. Citrus fruits and vegetables like orange, sweet lime, gooseberries, broccoli, potatoes, tomatoes, and some pure fruit juices are good sources of vitamin C.

D. Calcium

Calcium is needed for making baby's bones and teeth. Milk and milk products, fruits like banana, dry fruits like fig and apricot, almond, etc. are good sources of calcium. It is also supplied in tablet form by a doctor during and after pregnancy.

E. Omega 3 fatty acid

Bad Food

Food to be avoided or restricted during pregnancy:

1. Caffeine: Caffeine is naturally present in lots of food, like coffee, tea, chocolates, etc. It is also added in some soft drinks and energy drinks, certain cold and flu remedies. Higher level of caffeine may cause miscarriage and low birth weight baby. You do not need to cut caffeine out completely, but its use should not exceed more than 200 mg per day.

Caffeine contents in food and drinks:

- 1 mug of tea – 75 mg
- 1 mug of filter coffee – 140 mg
- 1 mug of instant coffee – 100 mg
- 1 can of cola – 40 mg
- 50 gm bar of plain chocolate - up to 50 mg

So, you can calculate your caffeine intake accordingly.

2. Smoking: Each cigarette contains about more than 4,000 chemicals. Every cigarette you smoke harms your baby in your womb by restricting necessary oxygen supply to your baby. So, your baby's heart has to beat harder every time you smoke. So it is a must to stop smoking. Both you and your baby will benefit immediately by clearing carbon monoxide (poisonous gas) from the body and bringing oxygen levels to normal.

Passive Smoking

What is passive smoking?

Passive smoking is the inhalation of smoke, called second-hand smoke (SHS) or environmental tobacco smoke by persons other than the intended active smoker.

Passive smoking increases the risk of still-birth by almost one-quarter (23 per cent) and is linked to a 13 per cent increased risk of congenital birth defects. The findings underline the importance of discouraging expectant fathers from smoking around their pregnant partners and warning women of the potential dangers of second-hand smoke both during pre-conception and pregnancy.

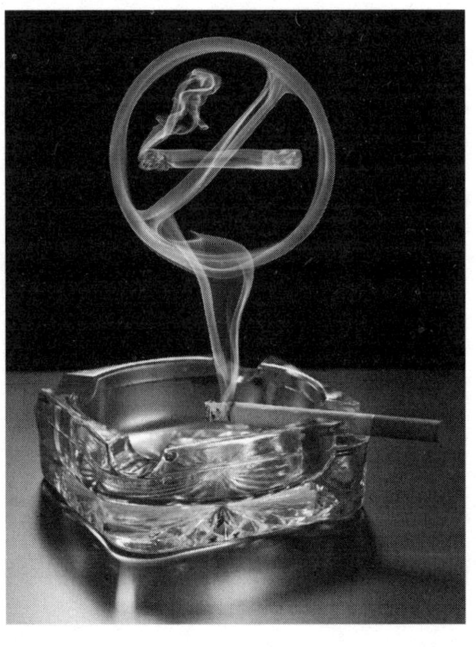

The researchers say fathers who smoke should be more aware of the danger they pose to their unborn child and that it currently remains unclear when the effects of the second-hand smoke begins. It is important to protect women from passive smoking both before and during pregnancy.

3. Alcohol: Whenever a mother drinks, alcohol passes from her blood to baby through placenta. The baby's liver is the last organ to develop fully and does not mature until

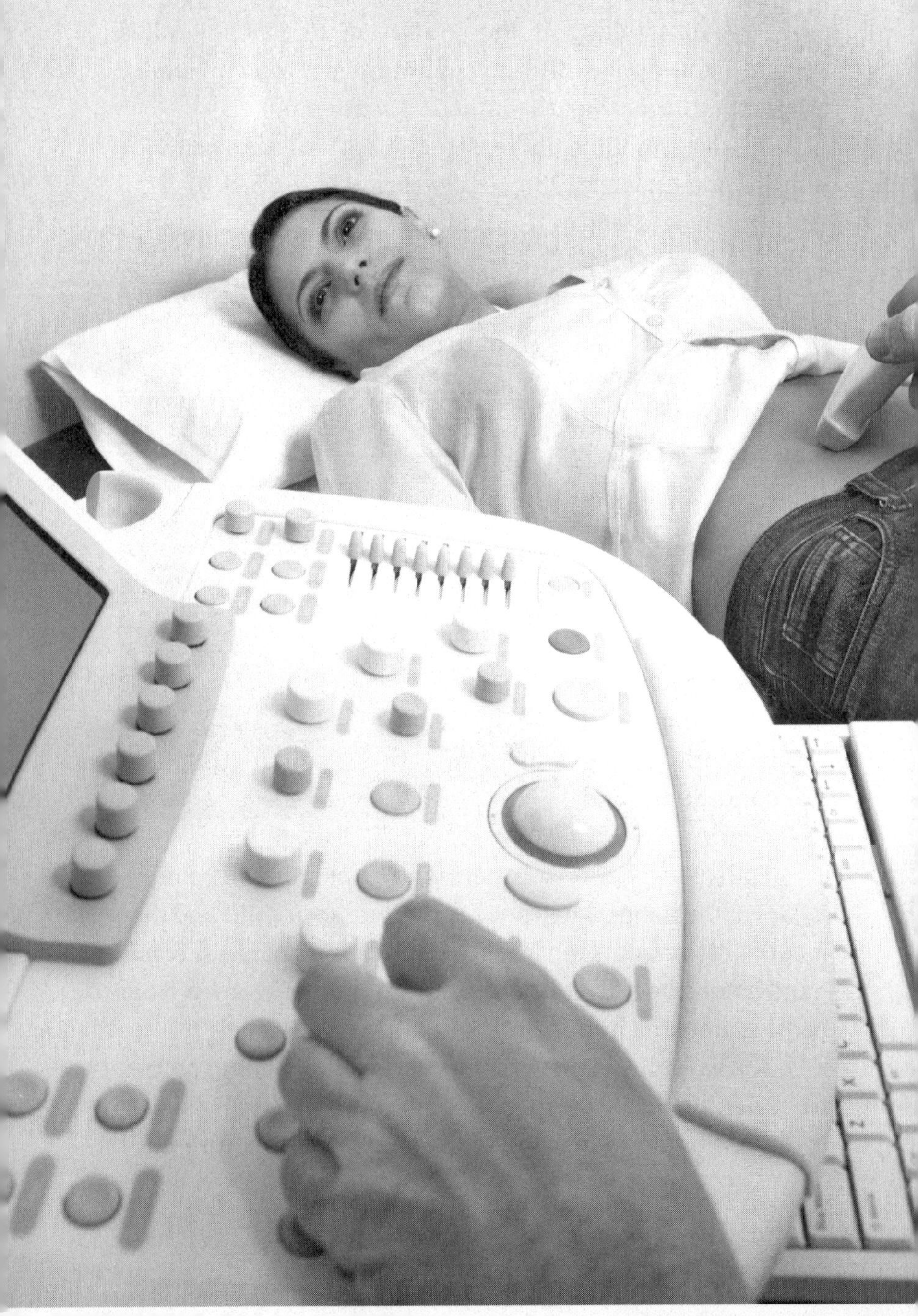

the later half of pregnancy. So, your baby cannot accept or digest alcohol like you can. In the early days of pregnancy, too much alcohol intake can result in miscarriage. Excessive intake of alcohol during pregnancy leads to some foetal abnormalities like restricted growth, facial abnormalities, learning and behavioural disorders.

4. Medications: It is preferred that whenever you are trying for pregnancy or are already pregnant, talk to your doctor regarding each medication that you are taking regularly. Your doctor will decide whether it is required to change it or stop it. Even some pain-killers are also harmful to your baby's health but some are safe. So, do not take any medicine without asking your doctor.

□

5

Antenatal Visits

Pregnancy, labour and birth of a child are important milestones in a couple's life. Regular medical care and understanding the unknown events during pregnancy can make childbirth an extremely enriching and joyful event.

Woman's health, behaviour, diet, habits and drug or illness affect the baby's development. Hence, you should take good care of your health and most important is to go for regular check-up with your doctor.

Minimum visits during pregnancy for rural non-affording patients

- At least 3 visits during whole pregnancy.
  - **1st visit:** Before 20 weeks (before 5 months)
  - **2nd visit:** 20-30 weeks (between 5 and 7 months)
  - **3rd visit:** 34-37 weeks (around 8-9 months)

In case of regular patients, it should be like this

- Routine schedule:
  - **Up to 13 weeks:** Every 15-20 days
  - **13 to 28 weeks:** Every 4 weeks
  - **29 to 36 weeks:** Every 15 days
  - **Thereafter:** Weekly
- In case of high-risk pregnancy:
  - **1st trimester up to 13 weeks:** Every 15 days or early whenever required

- **14-26 weeks:** Every 4 weeks
- **26-34 weeks:** Every 15 days or earlier whenever required according to sonography finding or high-risk factor
- **34 weeks onwards:** Weekly

What should be done in each and every visit?

1st visit: It should be after your missed period.

- Check for weight, blood pressure, pulse.
- Confirmation of pregnancy by urine test or blood test or by sonography.
- In sonography see for:
  - Presence of pregnancy.
  - Health of pregnancy.
  - Number of pregnancy.
  - Location of pregnancy (intra-or extra-uterine pregnancy).
  - GS (a bag of water in which pregnancy develops).
  - YS (Yolk Sac).
  - Foetal pole and Foetal heartbeat.

  It should be done only by TVS (internal sonography).
- Give folic acid supplementation. Give symptomatic treatment.
- Counselling about good health and nutrition.

2nd visit: 6-7 weeks

- Check weight, BP and physical examination.
- In sonography see for GS, YS, foetal number and shape, heartbeat, foetal pole, size and chorionicity.
- Advice for same medicines like folic acid, progesterone supplement if required and symptomatic treatment.
- Counselling about diet, health, travelling.

- Reassurance for pregnancy symptoms.
- Basic blood test for antenatal profile-Hb, Sugar, Blood Group, HIV, HBsAg, Thalassaemia screening.
- Give appointment for next visit.

3rd visit: 9-10 weeks

- Check weight, B.P. (blood pressure) and physical examination.
- In sonography, see for GS, YS, shape, heartbeat, foetal pole, size and chorionicity.
- Advice for same medicines like folic acid, progesterone supplement if required and symptomatic treatment.
- In case of high-risk pregnancy, give monitoring chart for blood pressure in case of hypertension, sugar chart for Diabetes Mellitus/Gestational Diabetes Mellitus (GDM).
- Counselling about diet, health, travelling.
- Reassurance for pregnancy symptoms.
- Prescribe appropriate medicine.
- Follow-up date for next visit after 15-20 days.

4th visit: 11-13 weeks

- Check weight, B.P. and physical examination.
- In aneuploidy scan, sonography (NT scan – scan for markers of certain chromosomal anomalies) to detect earliest abnormalities in foetus.
- Blood test like double marker for screening of Down's syndrome and other genetic syndrome.
- NIPT (non invasive pre natal testing) - it is screening blood test to rule out high risk of fetus for genetic chromosomal abnormality in high risk case.
- It is done between 9 weeks to 20 weeks of pregnancy.

- It is more sensitive (99%) than other non invasive tests (double marker, triple marker). Because it is done from foetal DNA (approximately 1 0%) present in maternal blood. There is no risk of miscarriage due to procedures as compared to invasive procedures (aminocentesis and chorion biopsy etc).
- For this test, maternal blood is collected by special kit, then fetal DNA is seperated from the sample and test is done from this fetal DNA
- OS tightening if required in high-risk pregnancy with bad obstetric history (recurrent pregnancy loss) or in multiple pregnancies.
- CVS (Chorionic villus sampling) in case of prior genetic disease or significant foetal history of genetic disease or higher risk factor in present pregnancy.
- Continue same medicine. After 13 weeks add iron, calcium, uterine relaxant, if advised, and protein powder supplementation.
- Tetanus vaccine – first dose.

5th visit: 16-18 weeks

- Check weight, B.P. and physical examination.
- In sonography see for foetal growth, heartbeat, placenta location, cervical length, liquor.
- Blood test for haemoglobin, sugar level, triple marker that is screening test for Down's syndrome and other genetic syndromes.
- Amniocentesis if there is high-risk for Foetus or any family history of genetic disease, previous sibling affected with genetic disease.
- In pregnancy with hypertension, blood pressure-monitoring chart.

- In pregnancy with diabetes, sugar chart, diabetic diet, etc.
- In pregnancy with thyroid disease, recheck thyroid hormone level and medicine accordingly.
- In medicines, continue iron, calcium, uterine relaxant and protein powder supplementation.
- Counselling for proper diet, nutrition, health.
- TT vaccine if not given previously.

6th visit: 20-22 weeks

- Check weight, B.P. and physical examination.
- Generally, it is a period of 3D-4D anomaly scan intended to detect anomalies in foetus, foetus, echo etc., and cervical length, uterine Doppler.
- In pregnancy with Hypertension -Blood Pressure monitoring chart
- In pregnancy with Diabetes – Sugar chart, Diabetic diet etc.
- In pregnancy with Thyroid disease – recheck thyroid hormone level and medicine accordingly.
- Continue same medicine.
- Counselling for proper diet, nutrition, health.
- Counselling about stem cells preservation.
- Counselling about where to deliver.
- Tetanus vaccine 2nd dose.

7th visit: 26-28 weeks

- Check weight, B.P. and physical examination.
- Look for growth of foetus, cervical length, placenta, liquor, Doppler screening.
- Same blood pressure chart, sugar chart in respective patient.
- Counselling about nutrition, health.
- Injection of steroids for foetal lung maturity.

8th visit: 30-32 weeks

- Check weight, B.P. and physical examination.
- Look for growth of foetus, cervical length, placenta, liquor, Doppler screening.
- Blood test like haemoglobin, sugar test.
- HBA1C (average sugar level of 3 months), thyroid profile in a high-risk patient.
- Injection of anti-D in case of Rh-negative.
- Same blood pressure chart, sugar level in the patient.
- Continue same medicine.
- Counselling about nutrition, health.

9th visit: 34-36 weeks

- Check weight, B.P. and physical examination.
- Look for growth of foetus, cervical length, placenta, liquor, Doppler screening.
- Same blood pressure chart, sugar chart in the patient.
- Continue same medicine.
- Counselling about nutrition, health.

□

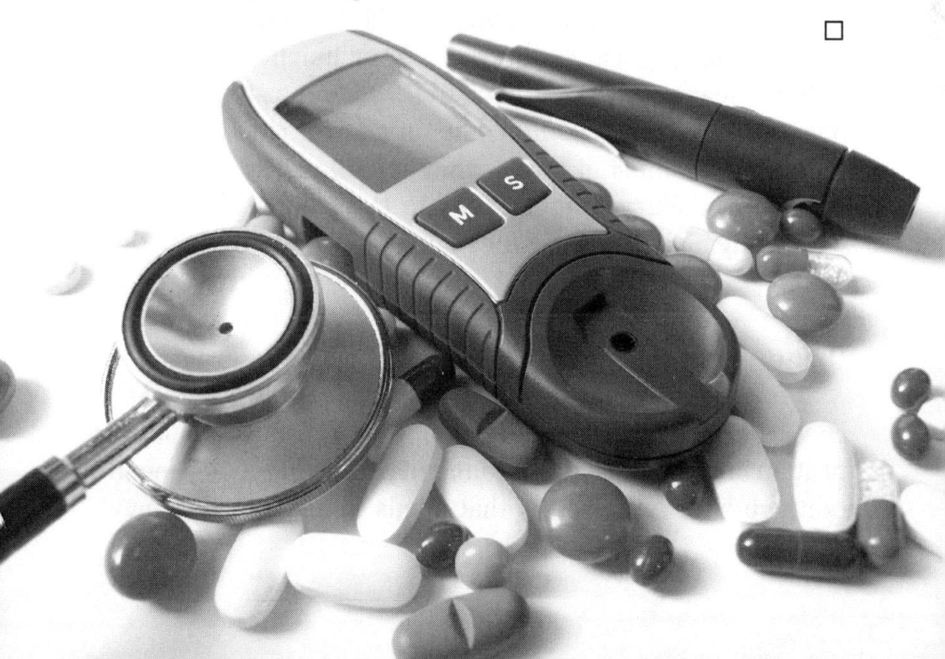

6

Blood Tests and Ultrasound Scans During Pregnancy

When the urine pregnancy test is positive, it is just the beginning of the tests and scans you will be undergoing during your pregnancy.

During your pregnancy, you will be offered a range of tests, including blood tests and ultrasound baby scans. These tests are designed to help make your pregnancy safer, to check and assess the development and well-being of you and your baby, or to screen for particular conditions.

Weight and height

You will be weighed at your booked appointment, and then regularly during your visits. Your height and weight will be measured so that your BMI (body mass index) can be calculated. Most women gain on an average 10-12.5 kg in pregnancy, most of it after they are 20 weeks' pregnant. Much of the extra weight is due to the baby growing, but your body also stores fat for making breast milk after the birth.

Urine

You'll be asked to give a urine sample at your pregnancy check-ups. Your urine is checked for several things, including protein or albumin. If this is found in your urine, it may mean that you have an infection that needs to be treated. It may

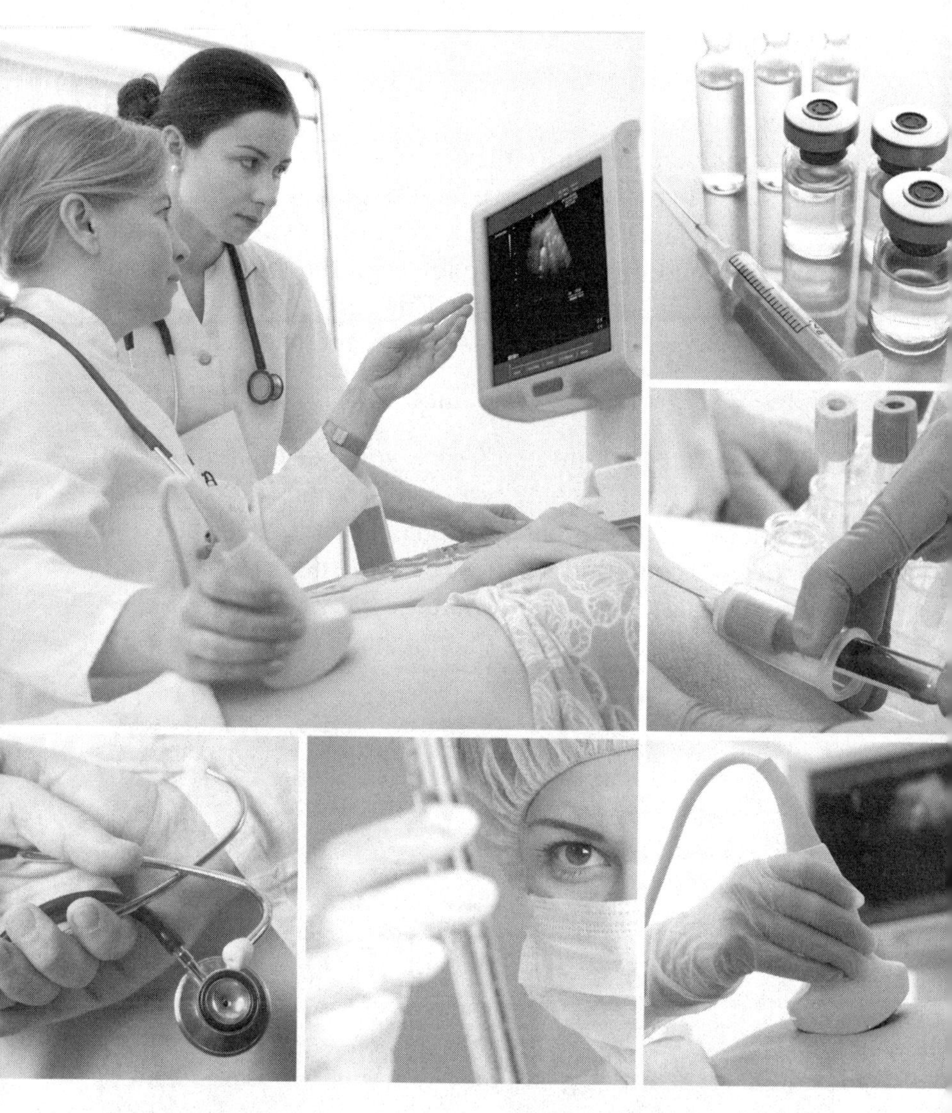

also be a sign of pre-eclampsia. Pre-eclampsia affects 10% of pregnancies, and can be life-threatening if left untreated. It can cause the pregnant woman to have fits, and affect the baby's growth.

Blood pressure

Your blood pressure will be measured at every antenatal visit. A rise in blood pressure later in pregnancy could be a sign of pregnancy-induced hypertension. It's very common for your blood pressure to be lower in the middle of your pregnancy than at other times. This isn't a problem, but it may make you feel light-headed if you get up quickly.

Blood tests

As part of your antenatal care, you'll be offered several blood tests. Some are advised to all women, and some are advised only if you might be at risk of a particular infection or inherited condition. All these tests are done to make your pregnancy safer or to check that the baby is healthy. Below is an outline of all the tests that might be advised.

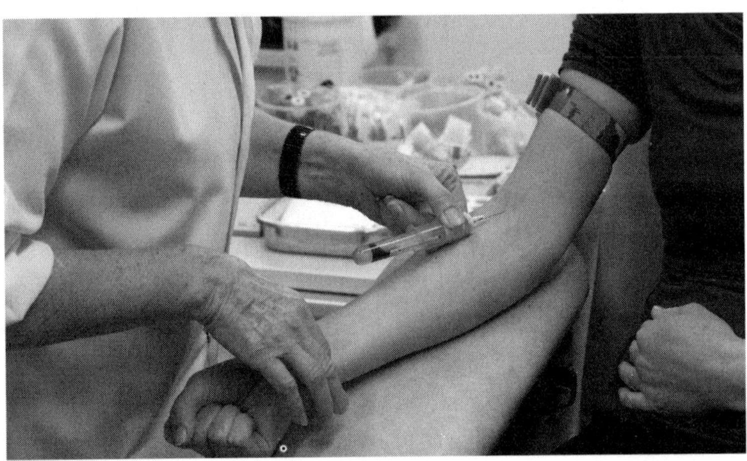

Blood group

It is a must to know your blood group whenever you become pregnant.

Anaemia

A full blood count, including haemoglobin and to check that you are not anaemic. Anaemia makes you tired and less able to cope with loss of blood when you give birth or face any bleeding episode. If tests show that you're anaemic, you'll be given higher than usual dose of iron and folic acid.

Infections

You may be advised tests for:

- *Susceptibility to rubella (German measles):* If you get rubella in early pregnancy, it can seriously damage your unborn baby.
- *Syphilis:* You may be tested for this sexually transmitted infection because it can lead to miscarriage and stillbirth if left untreated.

Hepatitis B: This virus can cause serious liver disease, and it may infect your baby if you're a carrier or you're infected during pregnancy. Your baby won't usually be ill, but has high chances of developing long-term infection and serious liver disease later in life. Your baby can be immunised at birth to prevent this infection. If you have hepatitis B, you may be referred to a specialist.

- *Hepatitis C*: This virus can cause serious liver disease and there is a small risk that it will pass on to your baby if you are infected. It cannot be prevented at present. If you're infected, you'll be referred to a specialist, and your baby can be tested after it is born.

- *HIV (human immunodeficiency virus)*: This is the virus that causes AIDS. HIV infection can be passed on to a baby during pregnancy, at delivery or after birth by breastfeeding. As part of your routine antenatal care, you'll be offered a confidential test for HIV infection. If you're HIV-positive, both you and your baby can have treatment and care that reduces the risk of your baby becoming infected.

Thyroid profile

Thyroid hormone levels are checked to detect any overt or subclinical hypothyroidism which can affect the baby if not corrected.

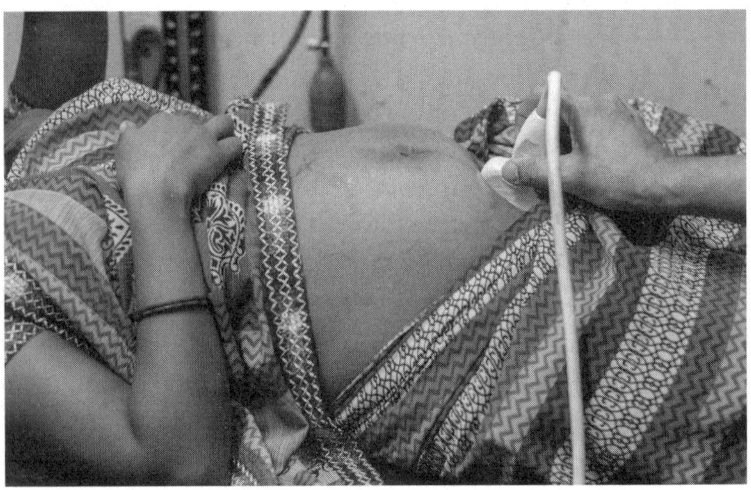

Another blood test is offered at around 28 to 30 weeks to recheck haemoglobin.

Gestational diabetes screening

You will also be screened for gestational diabetes between 26 and 28 weeks of pregnancy with a glucose screening test. It can be HBA1C or GTT.

HBA1C is the test that tells us your average sugar level of 3 months.

The GCT test is done in a clinic or medical laboratory and you will need to drink a sweet glucose drink, wait for one hour and then have a blood test. If your test shows that you may be at risk of having high sugar level, you will be asked to take a Glucose Tolerance Test (GTT). Many women who have a positive result will not have gestational diabetes.

Women with risk factors for diabetes may be offered the GTT first. For this test, you will need to miss breakfast and then have a blood test before having a glucose drink. You will then have blood tests at one hour and two hours after you have had the drink. If your test positive for gestational diabetes, you will be given advice on how to manage your pregnancy to keep you and your baby healthy and you will be referred to an endocrinologist and diabetes specialist for advice.

Ultrasounds

Women are offered three to four ultrasounds during a normal pregnancy, but some may require more for specific reasons. The ultrasounds that are offered to all pregnant women are:

First trimester ultrasound

A scan early in your pregnancy to check for:

- Presence and diagnosis of pregnancy
- Foetal heartbeat
- Number of babies

Repeat scans may be done depending on the possibility of a miscarriage or complications, or if you have a history of miscarriage.

11-13 weeks aneuploidy scan (Nuchal translucency scan)

The Nuchal translucency screening is done between 11 and 13 weeks of pregnancy. The scan is primarily a screening test for Down's syndrome and other chromosomal conditions, though the sonographer will also take some measurements and checks of your baby. The ultrasound is used to measure the thickness of the layer of fluid on the back of your baby's neck. This measurement is then combined with the result of a blood test which is done between 11 and 13 weeks and other factors, such as your age, weight and number of weeks of pregnancy to provide an individual risk assessment.

This result tells you if your baby has a low or high-risk of Down's syndrome. If you are considered high-risk, you will be offered genetic counselling to discuss your options.

3D-4D Anomaly Scan

This is a detailed ultrasound performed between 18 and 20 weeks of pregnancy, which screens for structural or physical abnormalities in the brain, heart, spine and other important organs.

You may also be offered other scans for medical reasons

Cardiac ultrasound (Foetal echo)

If you have diabetes, a family history of heart abnormalities, or a high nuchal translucency thickness, a cardiac scan (foetal echo) is sometimes performed around 22 to 24 weeks. A detailed examination of your baby's heart and connecting blood vessels is performed by an experienced sonographer with specific expertise in this area.

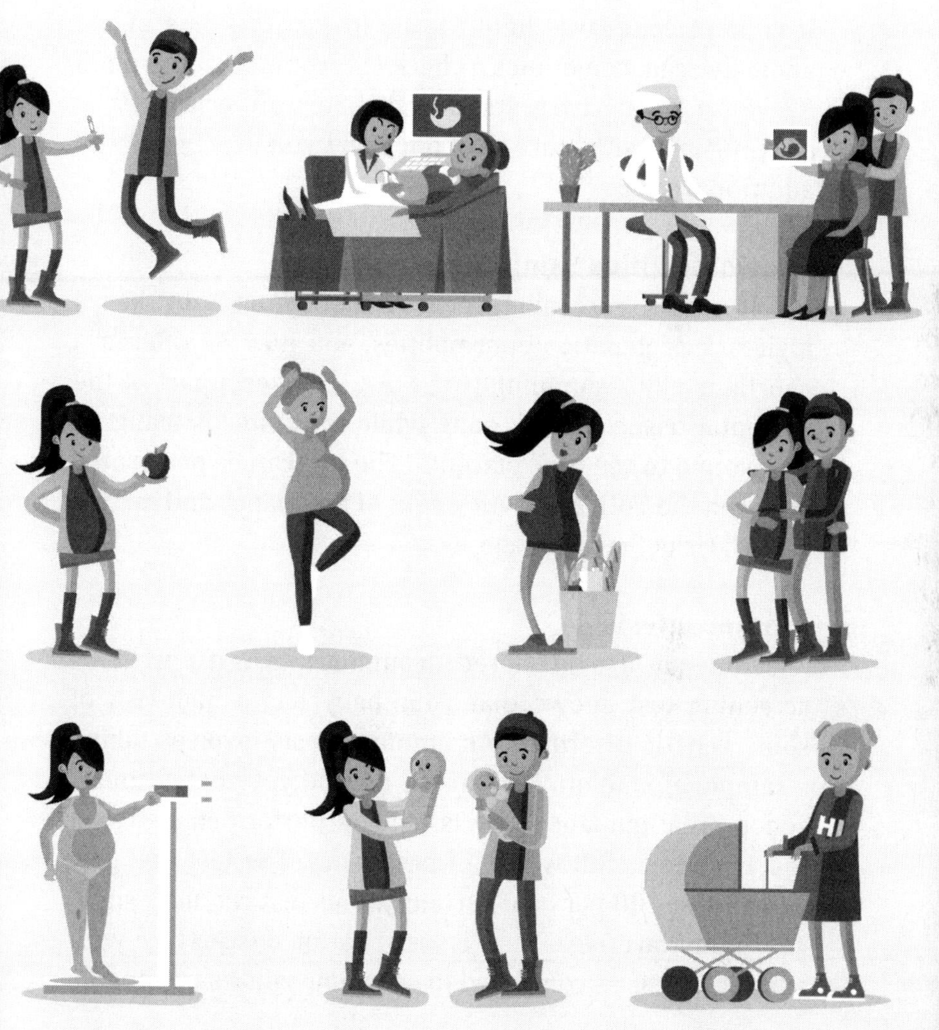
HI

Third trimester ultrasound (Growth monitoring)

If you have had complications in previous pregnancies or have developed a problem during this current pregnancy, you may be offered other scans in your third trimester. If your placenta was found to be low at the time of the anomaly scan, sometimes a check is recommended around 32 weeks. If you have gestational diabetes, pre-eclampsia or are pregnant with more than one baby, you may be offered additional scans.

Chorionic Villus Sampling (CVS)

If earlier screening suggests that your baby has a high-risk of genetic abnormalities, you may be offered a chorionic villus sampling (CVS). A CVS takes a part of the placental tissue. This is done while the tester is using an ultrasound to see your placenta. The test can be performed between the 10th and 14th weeks of pregnancy and carries a small risk of miscarriage.

Amniocentesis

You may also be offered an amniocentesis if a previous screening test shows that your baby has a high-risk of some genetic disorders. An amniocentesis involves taking a sample of amniotic fluid (fluid around your baby) under sonography guidance and is usually performed between the 15th and 18th weeks of pregnancy. The test will give you almost 100 per cent certainty. This test carries a small risk of miscarriage. There is less risk for miscarriage with amniocentesis as compared to chorionic villus sampling.

□

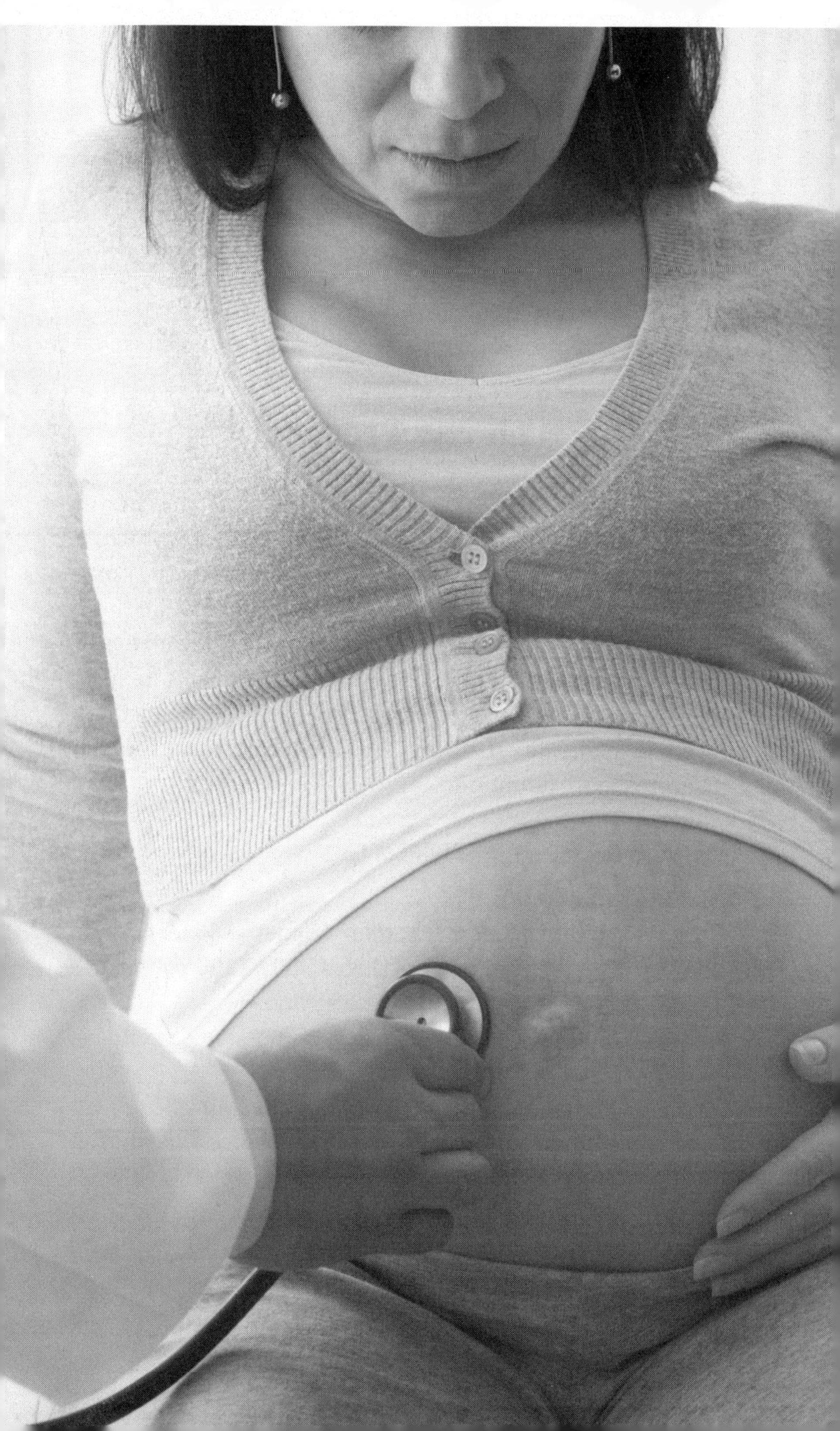

7

High-risk Pregnancy

Whenever there is increased risk to either mother or baby or both, it is a high-risk pregnancy. Risk factors for mother or baby may be existing before pregnancy or may develop during pregnancy. It is necessary to know all these factors so that pregnancy and delivery can be managed properly and both mother and baby can be taken care of.

In India, higher rates of maternal and foetal mortality are due to inability to diagnose them in early stages, which requires more attention.

Risk Factors

A. Maternal factors

1. Mother's height less than 1.5 metres [5 feet].
2. Mother's weight less than 45.5 kg [100 pounds].
3. Obesity.
4. Mother's age less than 20 years.
5. Mother's age more than 35 years.
6. Previous delivery by caesarean section.
7. Medical disorders existing before or during pregnancy like:
    - High blood pressure
    - Diabetes mellitus
    - Severe anaemia

- Heart attack
- Epilepsy
- Psychiatric disorder
- Kidney disorder
- Heart valve problem
- Asthma
- Rheumatoid arthritis
- Lupus, etc.

8. Drug use, alcohol or smoking addiction before or during pregnancy, medications like antidepressant, anticonvulsant drugs.
9. Mother having Rh-negative blood group.
10. Problems in previous pregnancy like:
    - Preterm labour
    - High blood pressure with edema
    - Convulsions
    - Retained placenta or post-partum haemorrhage
11. Infectious disease during pregnancy like:
    - HIV
    - Hepatitis C
    - Syphilis
    - Toxoplasmosis
    - Chickenpox
12. Breech presentation at full term in primigravida (first pregnancy).
13. Placenta previa (low placenta covering internal os)

B. Factors related to foetus

1. Possibility of congenital anomaly in ultrasound examination.

2. Foetal growth restriction or possibility of low birth weight.
3. Multiple pregnancy (twins, triplets, or more).
4. Past history of preterm delivery or foetal death in previous pregnancy.

These above, mentioned factors may be harmful to mother or baby or both. So, in such cases, proper antenatal, intra-natal and post-natal care of a mother and baby by a doctor (obstetrician and gynaecologist) and his experienced team is a must. Every high-risk pregnancy should be monitored and delivered at a tertiary centre well backedup with all technologies and NICU [neonatal intensive care unit]. Any maternal or neonatal complication can be taken care of and treated efficiently at such places.

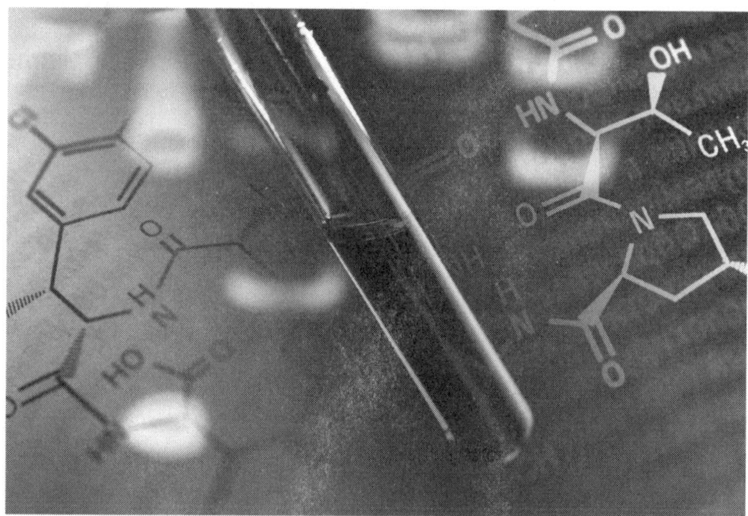

In many high-risk pregnancies related to neonatal causes, it may be easy to deliver mother at peripheral centre, but it may be difficult to deal with the requirements of the newborn. When it may require high quality and complicate immediate treatment it may not be available or possible at delivery centre. In certain cases, everything is smooth and normal, but the newborn may develop certain unexplained complications immediately after birth and parent may have to rush to tertiary centre for NICU but the condition of the newborn may not permit that much at the time. Immediate (initial 5 minutes after delivery) is the most critical period for a newborn and is the time to interfere for survival of baby.

If we analyse this situation, it is clearly necessary that it is better to transfer baby to well occupied experienced centre when it is in uterus (in-utero transport). If the baby reaches such a centre before delivery, it can be easily treated there after delivery.

If the pregnancy is high-risk and it is likely that the baby may need extra care and treatment. It is advisable to conduct such delivery at good, experienced and well-equipped centres where mother and baby both can be taken care of.

C. IVF pregnancy itself is a high-risk pregnancy

There are so many unexplained factors which might have caused infertility and contribute to high-risk pregnancy:

- Age
- Obesity
- Diabetes
- Hypertension
- Previous major abdominal/pelvic surgery

It is a difficult thing to get pregnant, and hence, any loss is much more important.

□

PREGNANCY

infographic about the prenatal development

Major blood vessels form

Formed neural tube from which will develop the spinal cord and spine

Embryonic

Upper limb bud forms

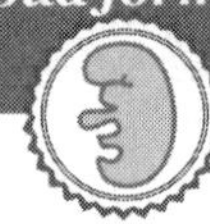

The embryo's skin is only one cell thick, this makes the skin transparent

Embryonic

Lower limb bud forms

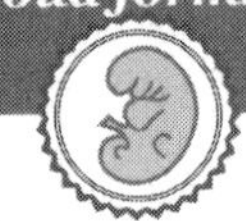

6 weeks pregnant. Size of 4 mm and a fertilized egg up to 25 mm.

Embryonic

Hand plate forms

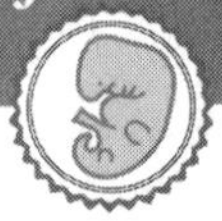

7 weeks pregnant. Size of 5–13 mm, weight 0,8 g

Embryonic

Webbed fingers and toes

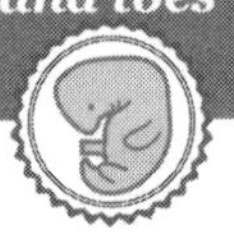

8 weeks pregnant. Size of 14-20 mm, weight 3 g

Embryonic

Fingers and toes separate

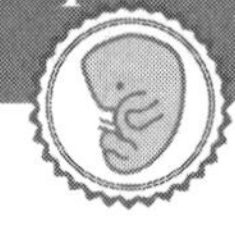

9 weeks pregnant. Size of 22-30 mm, weight 4g

Fetal

Differentiate by sex

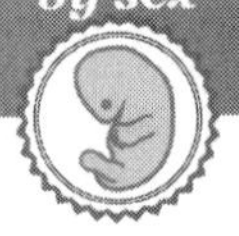

10 weeks pregnant. Size of 31-42 mm, weight 5 g

Fetal

Eyelids form

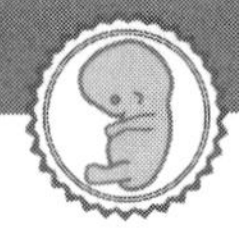

11-12 weeks pregnant. Size of 61 mm, weight 9-13 g, heart rate was 145

Fetal

Iris develops

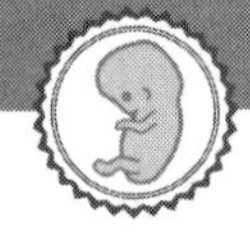

13-14 weeks pregnant. Size of 80-113 mm, weight 25 g

Fetal

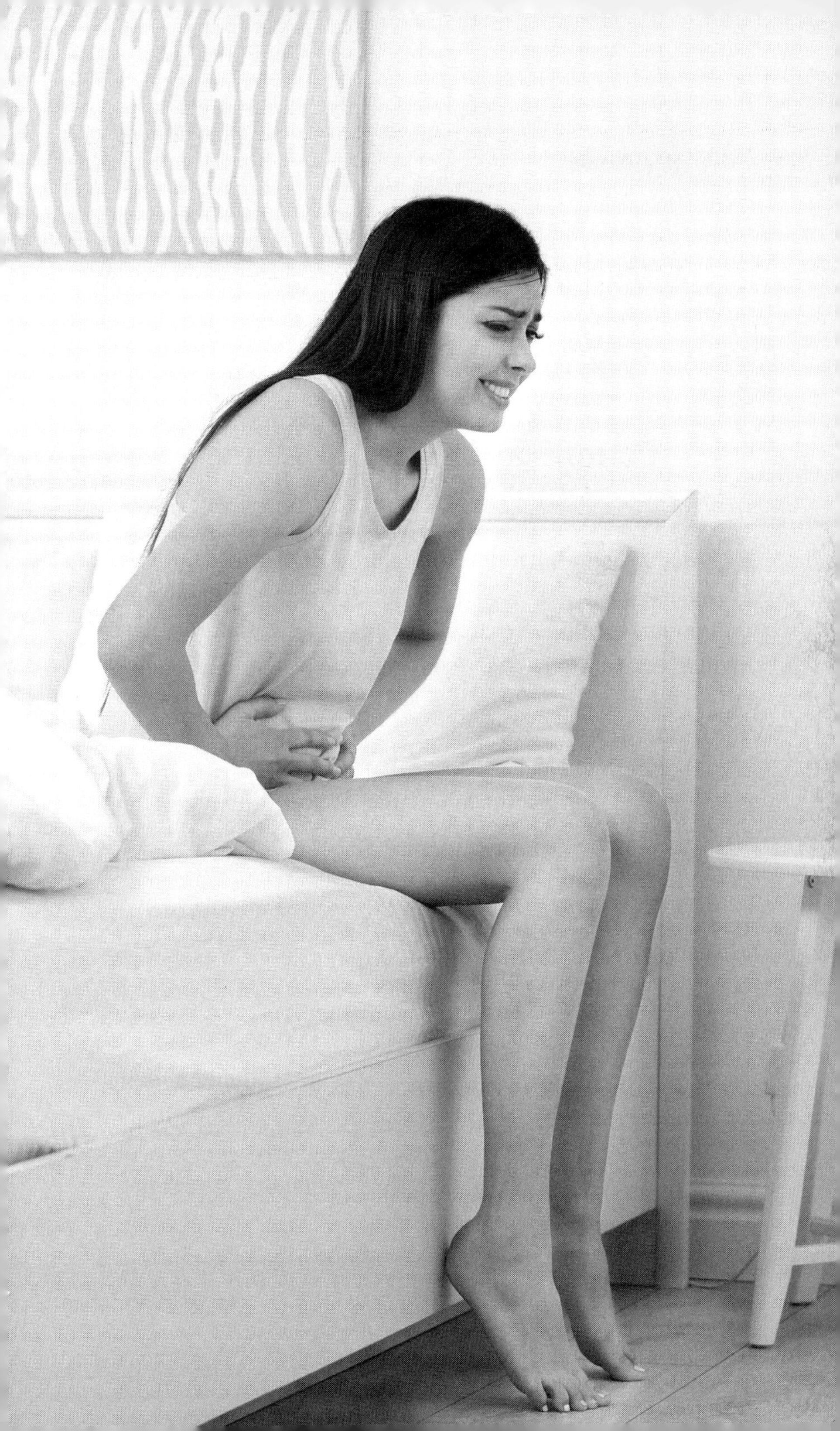

8

Complications and Warning Signs in Pregnancy

Most women have normal healthy pregnancy, but they have questions when we have to call doctors. These are some warning signs during pregnancy that we have divided according to each trimester.

1st trimester

1. *Vaginal bleeding:*
    - Some spotting is normal. But if heavy, bright red-coloured bleeding occurs, you have to contact your doctor.
    - It may be a sign of threatened miscarriage or ectopic pregnancy.
2. *Abdominal pain:*
    - If it is acute cramping, then it may be because of threatened abortion.
    - If it is sharp, then it may be a sign of ectopic pregnancy.
3. *Fainting spells:*

    If you have sudden fainting, then it may be a sign of ectopic pregnancy.
4. *Excessive nausea and vomiting:*

- It is common to have some nausea and vomiting during pregnancy.
- If it is severe and the patient cannot tolerate anything and it affects or interferes in the day-to-day activities and leads to weight loss, dehydration, dizziness, imbalance of electrolytes, then the doctor needs to be contacted immediately.

5. Fever more than 100°-101° F.
6. Leg/calf cramps or swelling on legs/severe headache.

As the pregnancy is a state of hypercoagulation, it may also lead to leg cramps, if it affects lower extremities and if it affects the brain, then it may lead to severe headache, but in case of severe headache, you have to check your B.P. because high B.P. may also lead to headache.

7. Exacerbation of underlying diseases, like thyroid, B.P., diabetes mellitus, asthma.

5 Warning signs of
PREMATURE !!!
1 Vaginal Bleeding
2 Hingh blood pressure,Swelling
3 Baby belly move less
4 Rupture of membranes
5 Abdominal stiffness
and longer and more frequent
Immediately see a doctor within 24 hours.

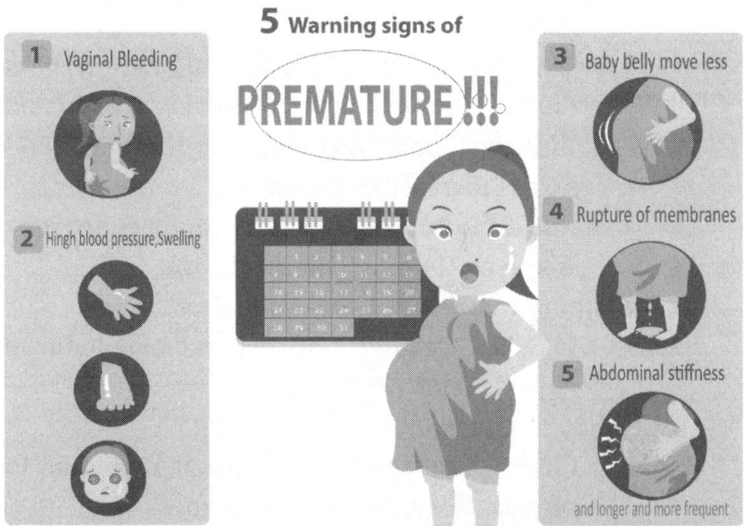

2nd trimester and 3rd trimester

1. *Vaginal bleeding:*
   - If it is in 2nd trimester, it is due to placenta previa.
   - If it is associated with pain in lower abdomen, it may be due to placental abruption, meaning that placenta separates from uterus.
2. *Severe nausea and vomiting:*
3. *Baby's/foetal movement, if it declines significantly, then you should worry:*
   - In general, there are at least 10-11 movements/ day.
   - But if you have less movements then first take some food or liquid and then lie on your lateral sides and wait for movement. If you do not feel any foetal movement, consult your doctor.
4. *Contraction in 2nd trimester:*
   - It is a sign of abortion/preterm delivery.
   - There are normal physiological Braxton Hicks Contractions which occur in every patient and these are unpredictable, non-rhythmic, and do not increase in intensity.
   - But if the contraction is 10 minutes apart or frequent, then consult the doctor.
5. *Blurring of vision, headache and heartburn:*
   - It is related to pregnancy-induced hypertension (PIH).
6. *Leakage of membrane:*
   - Clear water burst from vagina is due to breakage of amniotic membrane.
7. Fainting attack.

8. Fever more than 100°-101° F.
9. Swelling of legs, hands and face.
10. Severe backache.

Minor but common problems in pregnancy

Following problems are very common in all pregnancies, but they are not warning signs; all these are due to altered physiology.

- Frequency of urination
- Non-specific discharge without itching
- Heart-burn/constipation
- Mood swings/irritability due to hormonal changes
- Incontinence: passing of urine during stress, coughing and sneezing.
- Itching
- Leaking nipples-normal
- Nose bleed – common and if it is profuse and frequent, then consult ENT doctor.
- *Piles*: You have lump or swelling outside the anus.

□

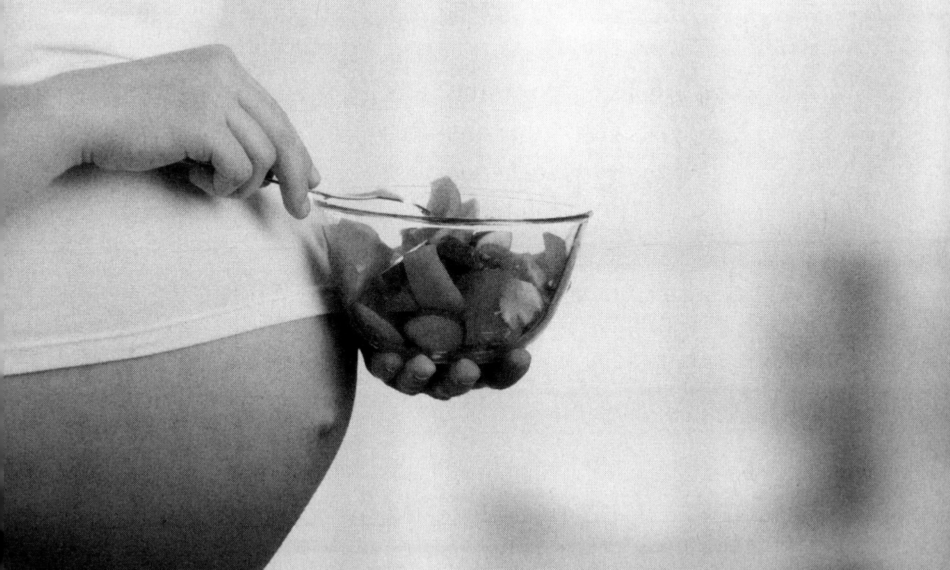

9

Health in Pregnancy

Pregnancy is the most wonderful and exciting stage of your life. You can make this phase even more fulfilling by planning in advance a healthy passage for both you and your baby. Attaining and maintaining good health is most important for a healthy pregnancy. First consult a specialist who can guide you through various stages of pregnancy.

There are some factors that will help you maintain good health in pregnancy, which are:

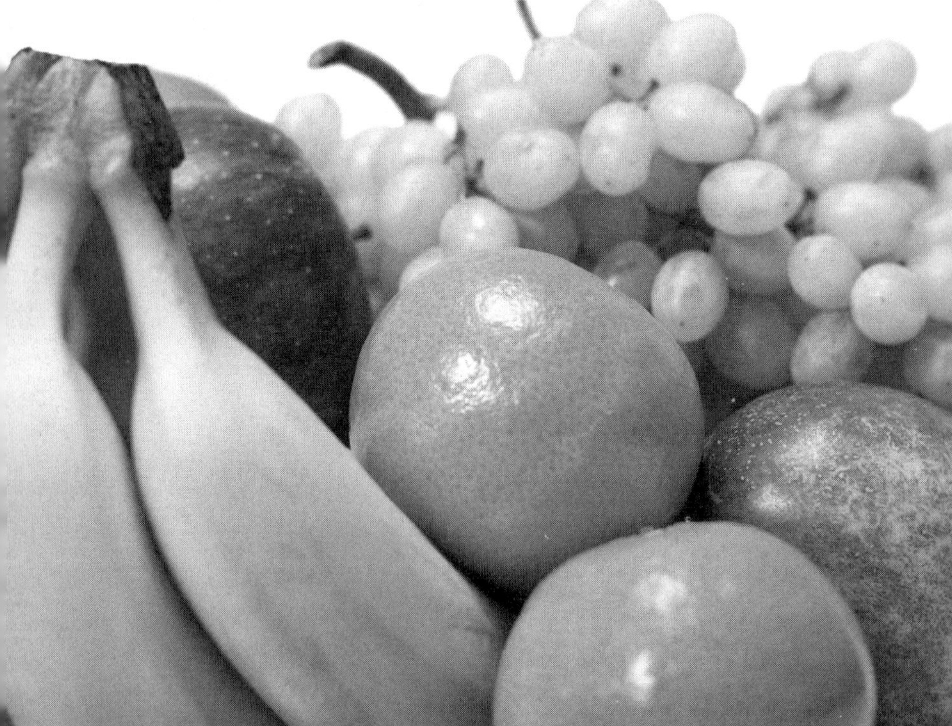

Diet Plan For a Pregnant Woman

Recommendation : 2175 Kcal (sedentary pregnant woman)
2525 Kcal (moderately active pregnant woman) to
3225 Kcal (very active woman). Protein 65 g/day

Early Morning	6:00am	Tea, Coffee orMilk	150 ml
Breakfast	8:00 - 8:30 am	Idly - 4 , Dosa - 4, Chapatti 4, Upma 4, Rice flakes upma, Sambar or Chuteny, Vegetable Curry and Egg or Paneer Dhokla	100 ml butter 100g flour 100g rava 4 cups 1 cups 1 no. 35 gm
Mid Morning	10:30 - 11:00am	Fruit salad, Veg salad, Buttermilk, Veg Soup or Non Veg Soup and Dry Fruits & Nuts	200 gm 1 cup 150 ml 150 ml 50 gm
Lunch	12:30 - 1:30 pm	Rice, Chapatti, Dal, Vegetables, Green leafy vegetable and Salad Non Veg, Soya bean, Paneer and Curd	3 cup 3 nos 1 cup 1 cup 1 cup 1 cup 75 gm 25 gm 50 gm 1 cup
Tea Time	4:00 - 6:00pm	Tea, Coffee, Milk, Ground nuts Sprouts or Bread Toast Veg Sandwich with cheese and Green gram dal payasam Bread pudding or Carrot halva	150 ml 100 gm. 1 cup 2 slices 1 piece 200 gm. 1 cup 1 cup
Dinner	8:00 - 9:00pm	Rice, Chapatti/ Bhakhri/ Thepla/ Paratha and Dal, Vegetables, Salad and Curd	3 cups 4 nos 1cup 2 cups 1 cup and 1 cup
Instructions	Note: Bed time warm milk - 150 ml / Note: 1 cup - 100 ml/g		
Include	Vegetables, salads, sprouts, veg soups Green leafy vegetables, Fruits Whole grains		
Allowance per day	Oil 3 - 4 tsp (15-20 ml) Sugar 3 - 4 (15-20m1) Salt 8g (1 ½ tsp)		

PREGNANCY NUTRITION

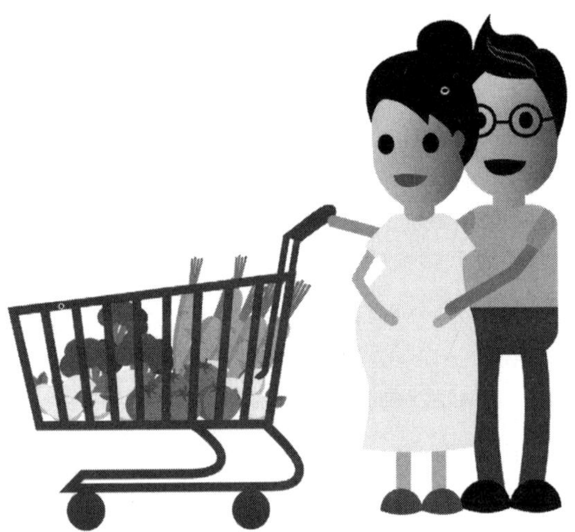

Average normal pregnancy weight gain

1st trimester : 0.5-1.8 kg during this period

2nd and 3rd trimester : 0.36-0.45 kg/week

Total weight gain : 11.5-16 kg

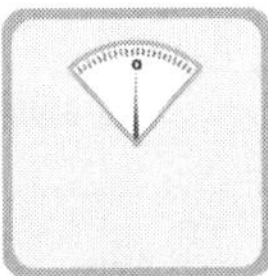

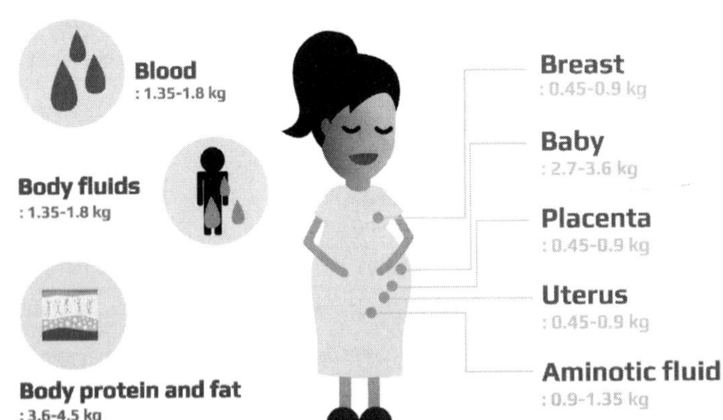

Attain a healthy weight

Proper weight maintenance can reduce the risk of complication due to underweightedness and obesity. Record the medical history of you, your partner and both families. If you find anything that raises concern, consult your doctor.

Manage your diet

Proper nutrition is vital for sustaining optimum growth and development of you and your baby. Take a balanced diet rich in proteins, vitamins and minerals, like iron, calcium, folic acid, etc.

Take prenatal supplements, especially folic acid in the first three months. This is vital for the brain development of the baby. Also take prenatal iron and calcium regularly.

Fluid

- Intake of optimum level of fluids is vital during pregnancy as it aids digestion, transport of nutrients and growth. It also prevents dehydration.
- Avoid excess sugar and salt as they may put you at a risk for hypertension and diabetes.
- Be sober and reduce caffeine intake. Increase fibre intake to avoid constipation.

Hygiene

Take care of your personal hygiene, keep your surroundings clean so that infections can be prevented.

Dental hygiene:

Dental care is important. If any problem is there, consult your dentist.

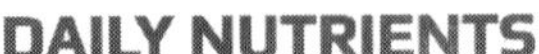

DAILY NUTRIENTS

Lorem ipsum dolor sit amet,
consectetur adipiscing elit

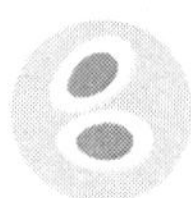

Protein
3 servings
(75 g total)
Lorem ipsum
dolor sit

Calcium
4 servings
(1200 mg)
Lorem ipsum
dolor sit

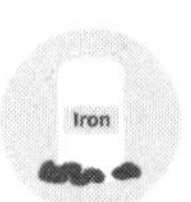

Iron
27 mg

Vitamin C
3 servings

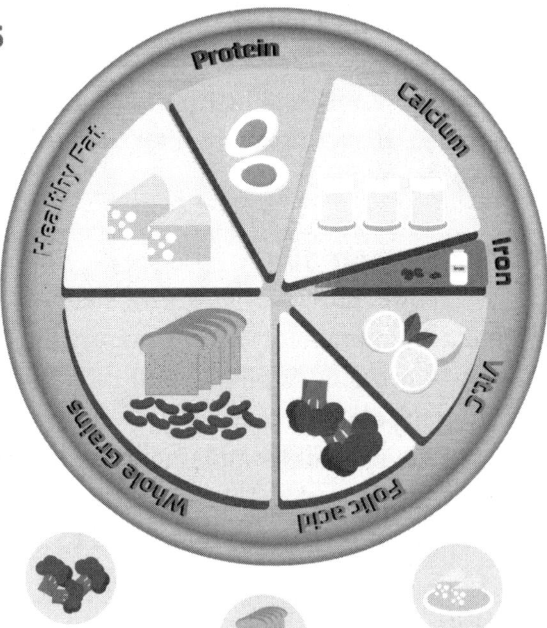

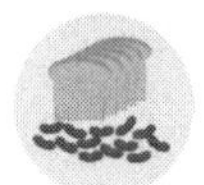

Folic acid
6-8 mg

Whole Grains
6 servings

Healthy Fat
4 servings

FOODS TO AVOID

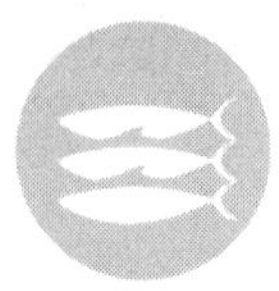

Shark, tuna
(High Mercury)

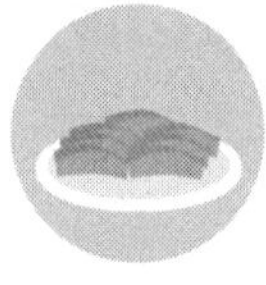

Raw/Undercooked
animal products

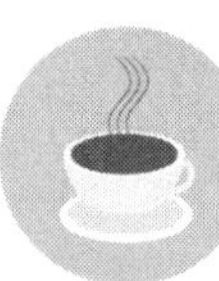

Alcohol
caffeine

Limit Cow's milk
high intake cause
fetal macrosomia

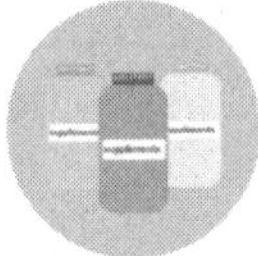

Unnecessary
supplements

High sugar added
food products

Bathing

Take daily bath and be careful against slipping.

Involve yourself in activities that can create positive vibes.

You should take proper rest and proper sleep for at least 8 hours at night and 2 hours at noon.

□

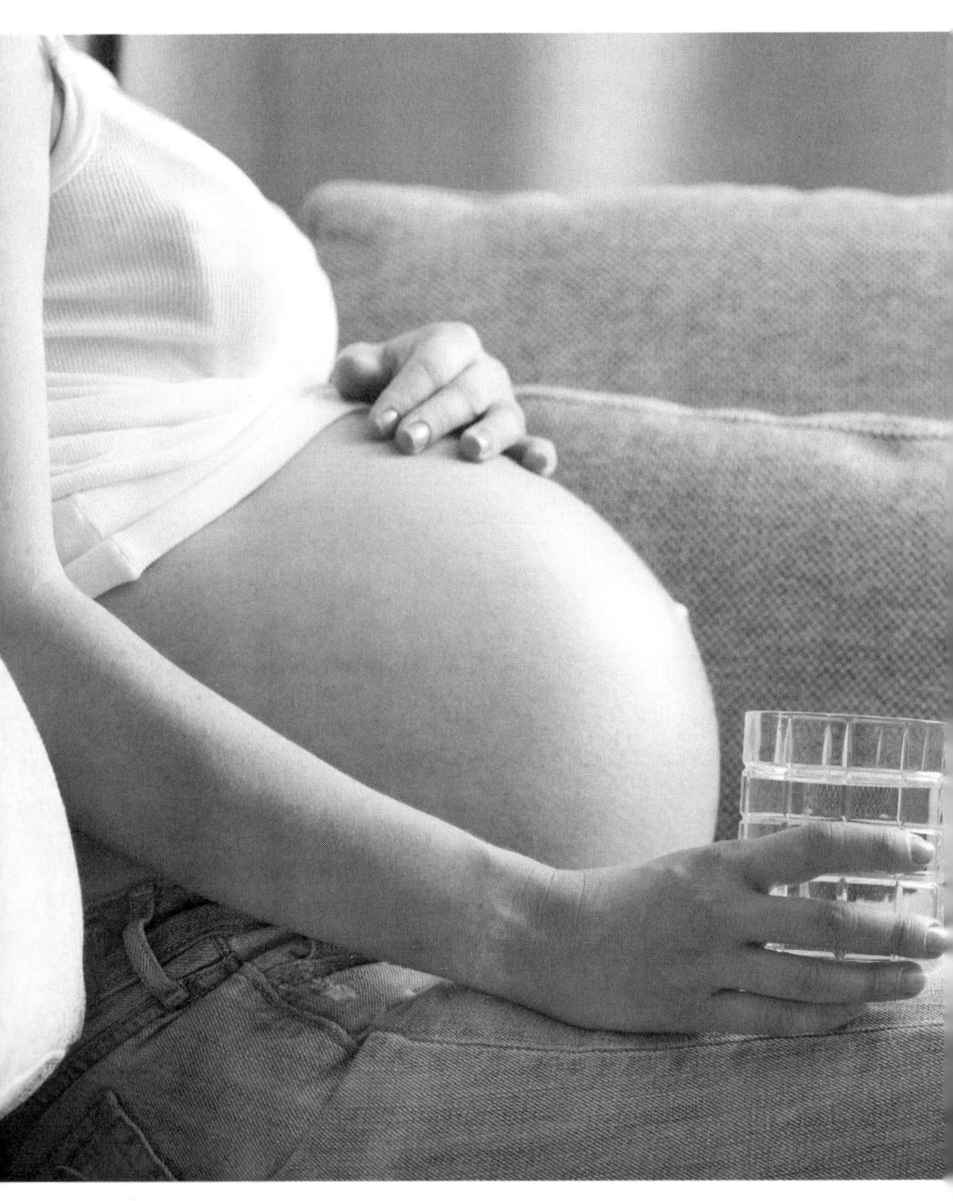

10

Precautions in Pregnancy

As soon as you see a positive pregnancy test, you may worry about what you can do, can eat, etc. There is no doubt pregnancy can be one of the most thrilling and most worrisome times in a woman's life. The most scary word for something that causes birth defect or harm to Foetus is teratogens that can be a drug, medicine, chemical, infections etc. Some warnings from friends and well-wishers are worth listening to, others are unproven facts.

Your doctor is the best person who can tell you about things which are harmful to your baby.

Diet precautions

Avoid excessive consumption of seafood and fish because some fish may contain high levels of mercury.

Caffeine : Some believe that caffeine can cause premature delivery and small for date or low birth weight babies. For details, refer to *Chapter 4: Food and Nutrition.*

Addictions: Avoid smoking and passive smoking as it can cause growth restricted babies and abortion. Alcohol in excessive amounts can cause birth defects known as foetal alcohol syndrome, so decrease intake or avoid taking alcohol.

Medicines:

- Avoid baking soda for heartburn but you can take soaked almond.
- Avoid taking brufen and other pain-killer medicines.
- Avoid laxatives and diuretics.
- Avoid self-medication and over-the-counter medicines.

Food handling:

- Avoid eating raw meat, fish or eggs.
- Drink only pasteurised milk. Avoid hot tubs and saunas, since they can cause overheating and affect development of the baby.

Pet handling:

- Avoid cat faeces, since it can cause toxoplasmosis (a parasitic infection).
- Reduce exposure to video display terminals, chemicals (if you are working in factories).

Things to do

- Sleep on your side. If possible, take 1-2 hours' nap in the afternoon.
- Use a step stool to reach high shelves.
- Drink plenty of fluids/water.
- Avoid stress.
- Adjust your car seat to accommodate your changing shape.

Things not to do

- Do not hold your breath while lifting weights.
- Avoid lifting heavy loads.
- Do not sit for long periods or change position when you feel uncomfortable.

- Take a stretch break.
- Do not clean pets and do not do gardening without wearing gloves.
- Do not strain for bowel movement.
- Do not overexert. If you feel short of breath, take rest.

Travel during pregnancy

As long as your pregnancy is free of any complication or concern, it is safe to travel most of the time during the early phase of your pregnancy. In later part of your pregnancy, you should travel after taking advice of your doctor.

You can travel safely at any time during the pregnancy if there are no complications in your pregnancy and is comfortable to you.

Now you have a question regarding mode of transportation.

Choosing the perfect mode of travel.

You should choose your mode of travel wisely. Choose the one in which you are most comfortable and able to complete your journey without discomfort.

Travelling by road

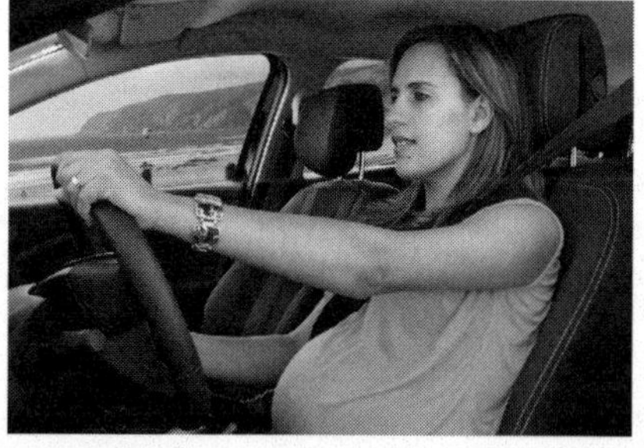

Road travelling can leave you exhausted. Hence, choose a vehicle that reduces the travel time as well as makes your journey less stressful. Cars are always better than buses due to the fear of jerks and bumps on the roads, though you must be very careful even in a car. Keep your seat belt well strapped to avoid sudden jerks and jolts. Keep a safe distance from the dashboard to avoid hitting it. Try to avoid front seat to prevent injury in cases of sudden jerks.

Tips for a safe road travel

Seat belt: The seat belt should be worn close to lower belly to avoid undue pressure on your tummy.

Snacking: Healthy and nutrient snacks on the way help prevent nausea during the first trimester and keep up your level of energy.

Relaxing: Make sure you get down for a stretch and walk for a few minutes after every hour or two to keep the blood circulation going smoothly in the body.

Comfort: A pillow can be carried to support your back and for a comfortable position.

Doctor's advice: Consult your doctor before heading for a trip during pregnancy. Your doctor should be the one to decide whether or not you should consider travelling.

Travelling by rail

Train journeys are much safer than road trips as there are fewer incidences of sudden jerks and bumps. With less jerks and enough space to stretch and lie down, you can easily travel longer distances while changing postures and moving around.

You must make sure that you hold on to the railings while standing or walking around. Be careful at the time of boarding and de-boarding.

Travelling by air

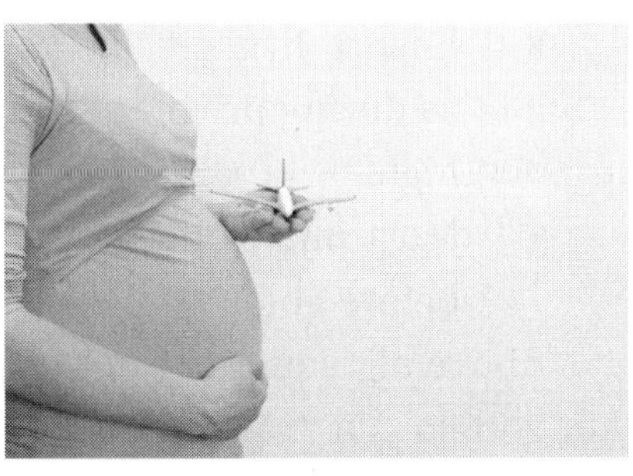

Travelling by air is the most comfortable and safe way. Get an aisle seat so that you can stretch and make yourself comfortable. Although, at higher altitudes, amount of oxygen gets diminished, you need not worry as the aircraft cabins are oxygen-pressurised.

In later part of pregnancy, for air travelling, you need to take your doctor's advice to confirm any high-risk factor.

Travelling by sea

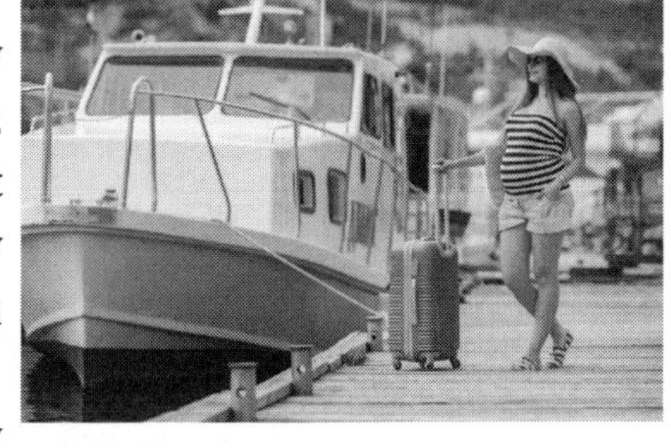

Sea travel is generally safe during pregnancy. The only demerit is that it elevates the intensity of nausea due to sea sickness.

There are few precautions that you must take while on a boat or a cruise:

- Get a cabin near the middle of the ship as it is less bumpy there.
- Always keep your medicines and reports handy.
- Go for hygienic and safe food in the cruise.
- Always keep light snacks with you.
- Consume light food frequently.
- Make sure you have at least the basic medical facilities on-board and proper medical care at the nearby shore.

- Ensure hygiene of the washrooms on the cruise as during pregnancy, the fear of infections is quite high.
- Most importantly, take the advice of your doctor before going on a trip.

Above all, you must not forget even for a minute that you should not travel alone. You have a companion who is much more fragile than you. So, one needs to take extra precautions while travelling during pregnancy.

Simple steps to take care of during travel

Avoid sitting for long hours. While travelling, make sure you get up to stretch and walk after regular intervals to avoid the fear of cramps and swelling. At the same time, wearing comfortable footwear also helps a lot to keep you agile and active.

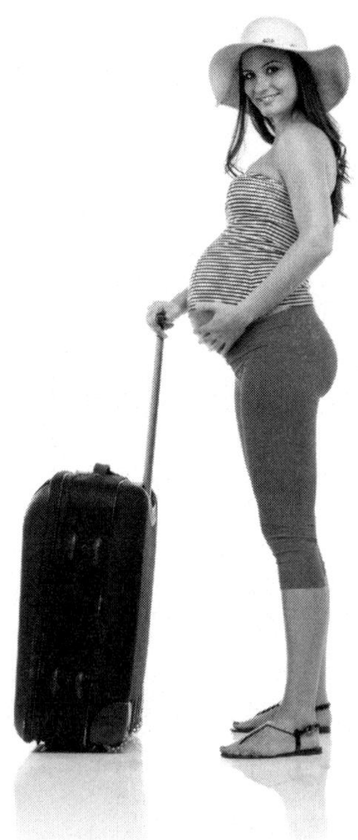

Do away with the nagging nausea. For most expecting mothers, nausea is bothersome during pregnancy. If you have a persistent problem of nausea, do not forget to keep an anti-nausea medicine prescribed by a doctor.

Follow the guidelines. There are certain things that

you should always follow while travelling. Like keeping a copy of your medical records handy for reference wherever you go or keeping the seat belt fastened below the belly while on the flight to avoid turbulence.

No carbonated beverages: Keep away from carbonated drinks, especially in the flight, to avoid abdominal discomfort and gas.

Eat frequently: Eat small portions at frequent intervals. Skipping meals should never be an option. If you don't like on-board food, carry small snacks from your home. While waiting at the airport or in transit, help yourself to some healthy snacks like dry fruits, protein biscuits or roasted nuts.

Fluid intake is a must: You should drink water, fruit and vegetable or mil- based beverages/juices to keep yourself hydrated.

Avoid air sickness: Mint, *saunf* and candies are very helpful to avoid air sickness during pregnancy. Carry some with you just in case you need them.

Avoid raw foods: Keep away from foods like uncooked eggs, salad dressings like Caesar's dressing or mayonnaise.

Pregnancy is all about taking care. And when you take care, you tend to enjoy the phase even more. Travelling during pregnancy is mostly due to unavoidable circumstances. Proper measures, if followed carefully, can keep your pregnancy healthy and safe even while travelling. Always remember, for these 32 weeks, you aren't alone. Whatever you do has an effect on the little one you are carrying along. Make sure you keep your baby safe and comfortable during travelling.

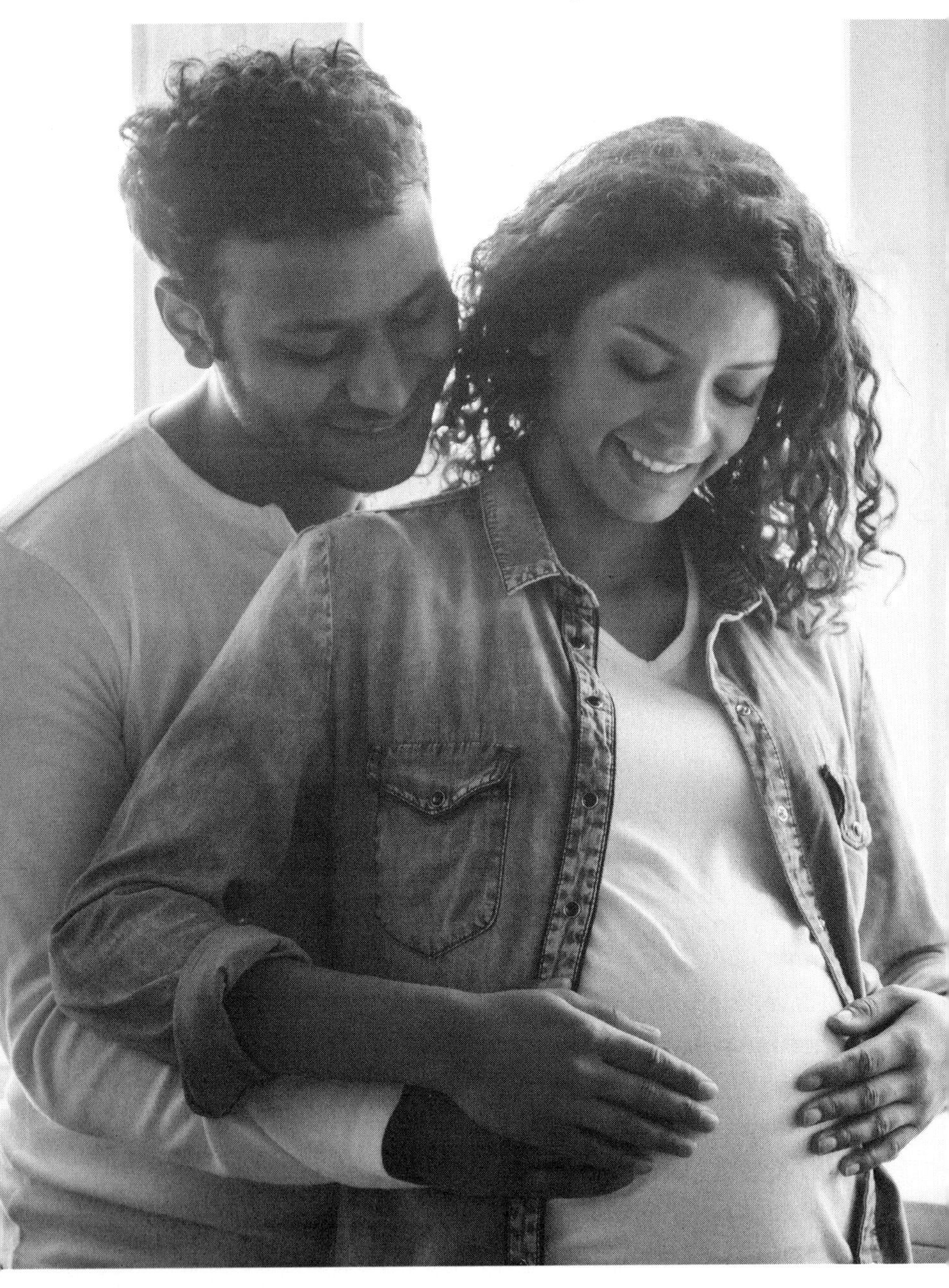

Sex during pregnancy

If you want to get pregnant, you have sex. No surprises there. But what about sex while you're pregnant? The answers aren't always as obvious.

Here's what you need to know about sex during pregnancy:

- At first, hormonal fluctuations, fatigue and nausea might sap your sexual desire. As your pregnancy progresses, weight gain, back pain and other symptoms might further dampen your enthusiasm for sex.
- Your emotions might take a toll on your sex drive too.
- As long as your pregnancy is proceeding normally, you can have sex as often as you like – but you might not always want to.

Avoid sex in following circumstances:

- A low-lying placenta (Placenta previa)
- If you have a history of miscarriage
- If you have taken fertility treatment
- You are above 35 years of age
- If you have spotting or bleeding in early pregnancy
- Abdominal pains or cramps
- Broken waters
- A history of cervical weakness and short cervix

You may also be advised to avoid sex during pregnancy if your husband has genital herpes. If you catch genital herpes for the first time during pregnancy, there is a small risk that it could affect your developing baby.

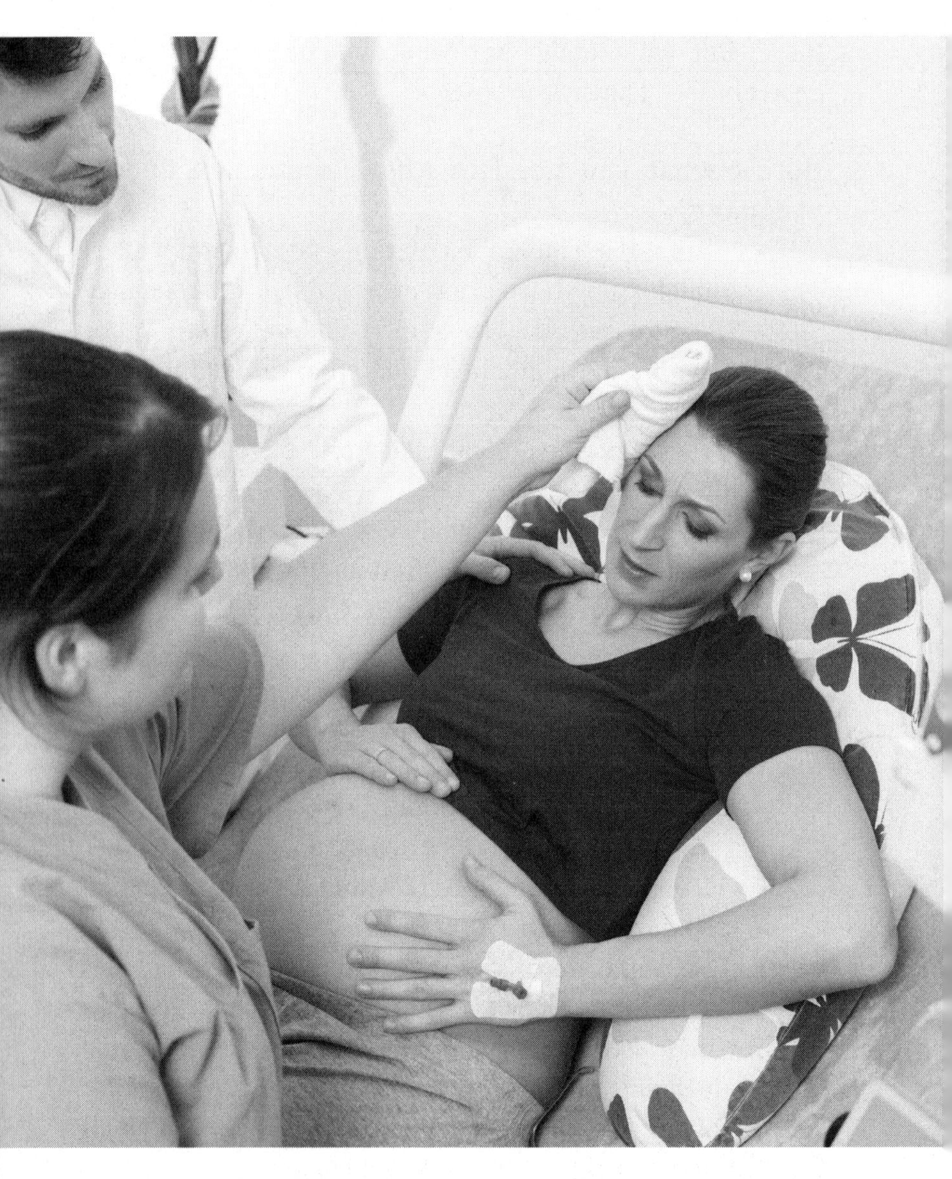

You won't hurt your baby by making love, even with your partner on top. The thick mucous plug that seals the cervix helps guard against infection. The amniotic sac and the strong muscles of the uterus (womb) also protect your baby. Though your baby may move about a lot after orgasm, it's because of your pounding heart, not because he knows what's happening or feels pain.

LDRS (labour delivery recovery suite), is a new concept for a woman who goes through labour delivery and recovery in one bed in the same private room with members of her family present (if she wishes).

□

11
Where to Have the Baby?

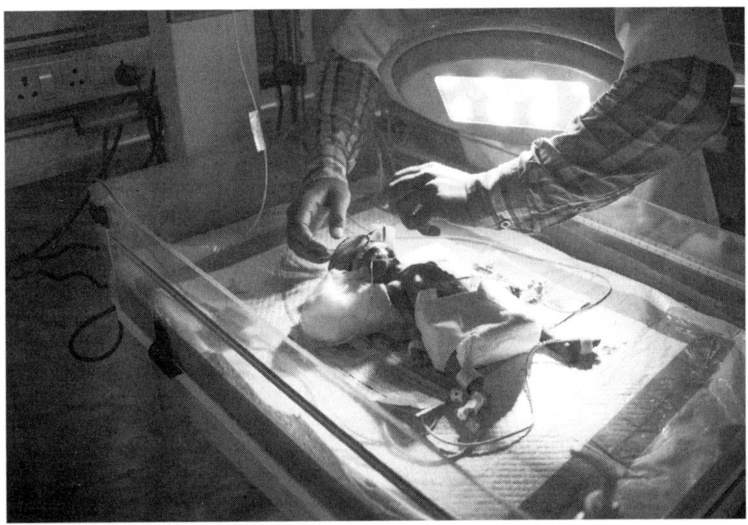

Early in your pregnancy, when you are deciding about your maternity caregiver, it is also important to make a thoughtful decision about where you plan to give birth.

Main consideration for choosing place of birth

- The care in the hospital should be the best available in the town or area.
- The staff should be committed and able to provide you with lots of support and comfort.
- Individualised care is given for you and your baby.

Facilities that you should look for in the hospital or nursing home

1. Separate labour room.
2. 24 hours availability of gynaecologist, anaesthetist and pediatrician.
3. Committed staff who are well versed in dealing with pregnant patients.
4. Availability of blood bank nearby.

These are for any woman without any pregnancy complications and a normal full term healthy pregnancy.

Other considerations are

- Are private rooms available?
- Does it have a neonatal resuscitation and initial care facility if baby has serious problems?
- Can the baby stay in the room with the mother?
- If pregnancy is complicated, you should consider hospitals with good operation theatres.
- Team of doctor (gynaecologist, anaesthetist, and pediatrician), neonatal ICU (NICU) and maternal intensive care unit with good experience of handling similar high-risk patients.

□

12

Emotions and Bonding Between Mother and Foetus

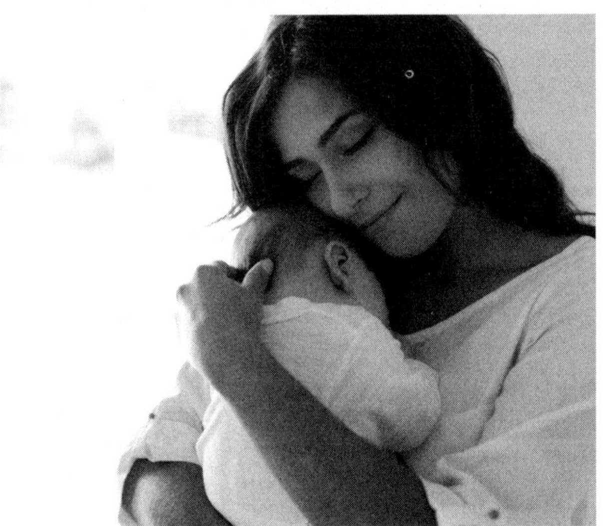

The baby is a living being from the time of conception and reacts to the environment in the mother's womb. Therefore, the physical condition, emotion and food intake of a mother are all factors that affect the baby.

Mothers who are serene and calm with little stress, while pregnant, will have a child that is calm and happy. People believe it helps to play soothing music to the baby, whilst it is in the womb. It may help if the mother takes relaxation classes to relieve tension and fatigue.

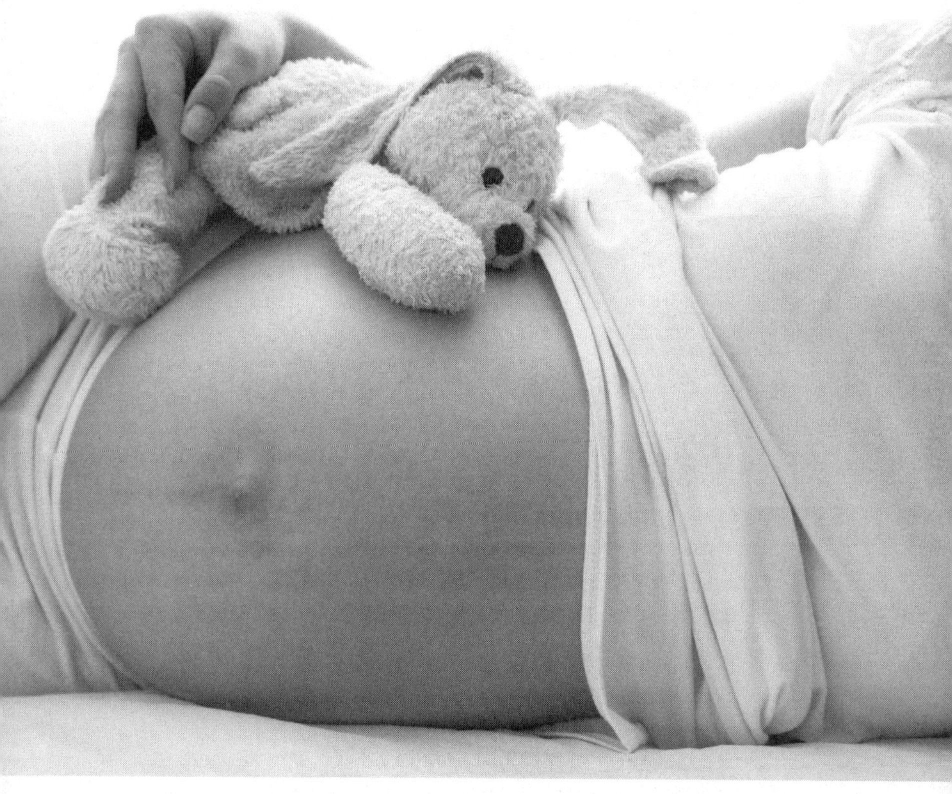

With the right kind of help, mother and child gradually bond. If the mother has a good experience in labour, she finds bonding with her baby easier resulting in the child being happier and settled. Attend prenatal classes and learn breathing and relaxation techniques.

After the baby is born, try and sleep whenever you can, as your nights may be disturbed at first. Try and relax, take time to play with, talk to and hug your baby. In other words, take time to bond with the baby and interact. Never feel that you are a failure because you cannot cope; be open with your family and your friends.

□

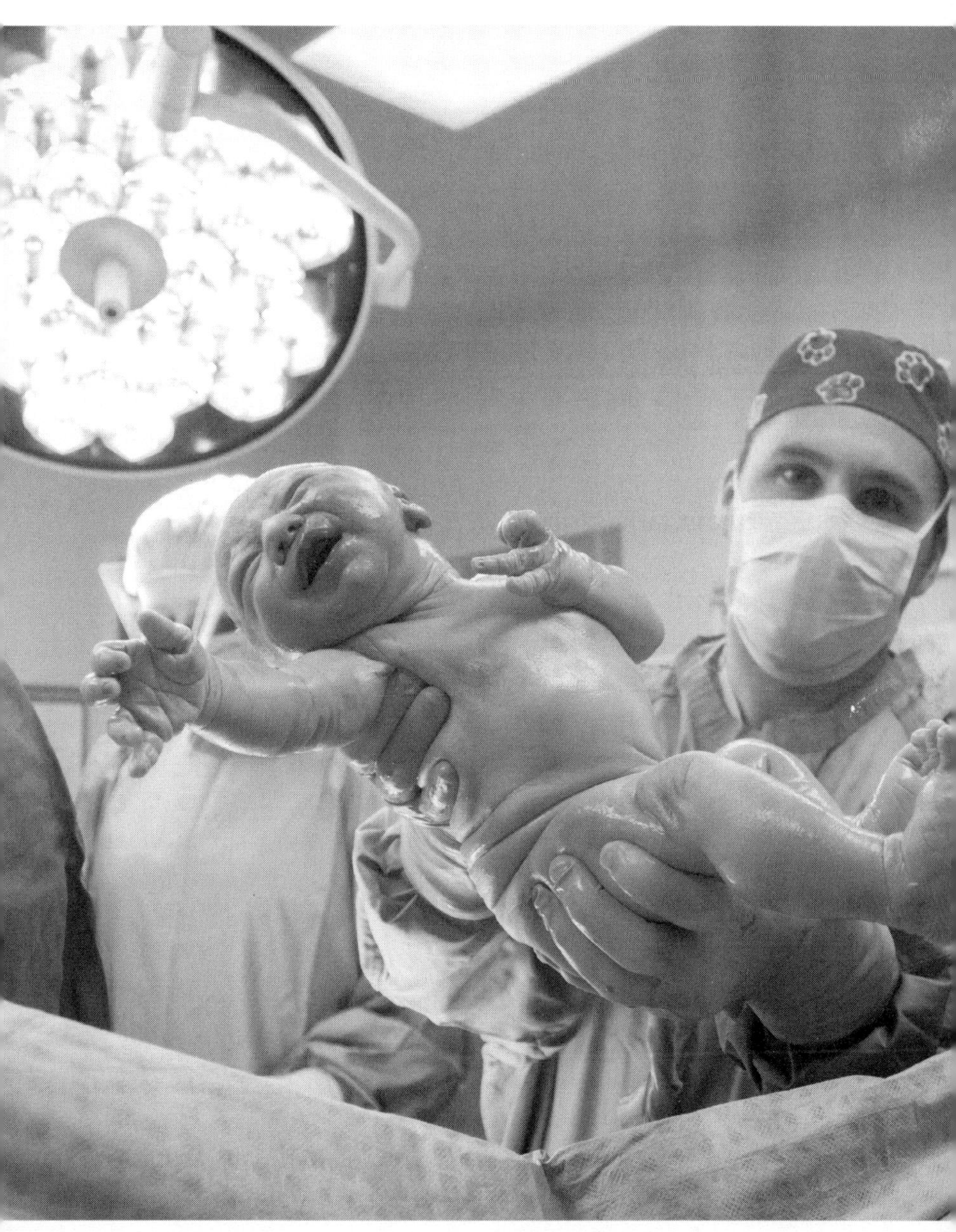

13
Labour and Childbirth

Starting labour pain and going into labour is exciting but may be difficult to manage if you are not prepared well in advance to welcome your baby. Knowing about all the stages and what to expect may help you feel more comfortable and in control of the situation.

Get ready in advance

- You should get ready at least 4 weeks before your due date.
- Keep your bag ready, including 2-3 loose, comfortable outfits, 2-3 supportive (large) bras, nursing bras, a kit with toothbrush, toothpaste, towels, front opening gown or night dress, clean clothes and nappies for the baby, sanitary napkins for you, a coverlet for the baby, phone charger, camera, etc.
- Think of mode of transport, whenever labour pain starts, to reach the hospital. Keep a vehicle ready.

Labour signs

It is very unlikely that you may mistake labour pains. However, following are some of the signs:

- Backache with heaviness in lower abdomen similar to what a woman feels during her periods.
- Abdominal pain with tightness of abdomen at regular intervals. (i.e., uterine contractions). During contractions, uterus tightens and relaxes at regular intervals. Intensity and frequency of contractions increases as time passes.
- The 'show', the mucous plug in cervix which helps seal the uterus during pregnancy, comes out of the vagina as labour starts. It is minimally blood stained and sticky and is called the 'show'.
- Rupture of water bag. The bag of water surrounding your baby may break during labour or before labour pain starts. It may be a sudden gush of water or little trickle minimally blood-stained fluids.

How labour progresses

There are three stages of labour. In the first stage, cervix gradually opens up. In the second stage, baby is pushed down in vagina and born. In the third stage, placenta gets separated from wall of uterus and comes out of vagina.

After vaginal birth

Immediately after birth, skin-to-skin contact with your baby is important as it helps in bonding and your baby will also like it.

In case of episiotomy (incision given by a surgeon on perineum), or perineal tear stitches will be taken. In such cases avoid squatting and sitting cross-legged for 7 to 10 days according to your doctor's advice.

Caesarean section (Abdominal birth)

There are certain situations and indications where the safest option to deliver the baby is by caesarean section. A baby is delivered by cutting through your abdomen and uterus. The cut is made across the lower abdomen, just below the bikini line.

LDRS (labour delivery recovery suite), is a new concept for a woman who goes through labour delivery and recovery in one bed in the same private room with members of her family present (if she wishes).

□

14
Preparation for Breastfeeding

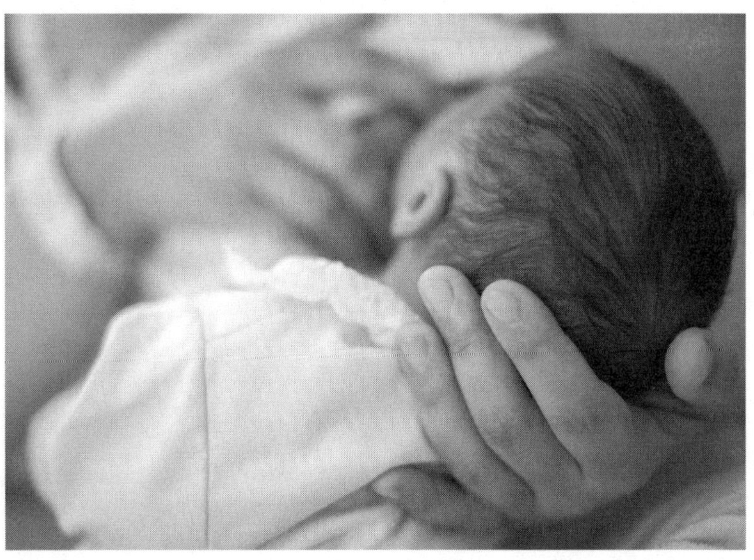

Breast milk is THE BEST and COMPLETE MEAL for a baby. During pregnancy, many physical changes take place in a mother's body, like abdomen, thighs, including breasts. These changes are physiological, but it is essential for a to-be-mom to know about these changes.

As the pregnancy progresses, both breasts start increasing in weight and size due to fat deposition and development of milk ductules as a part of preparation for

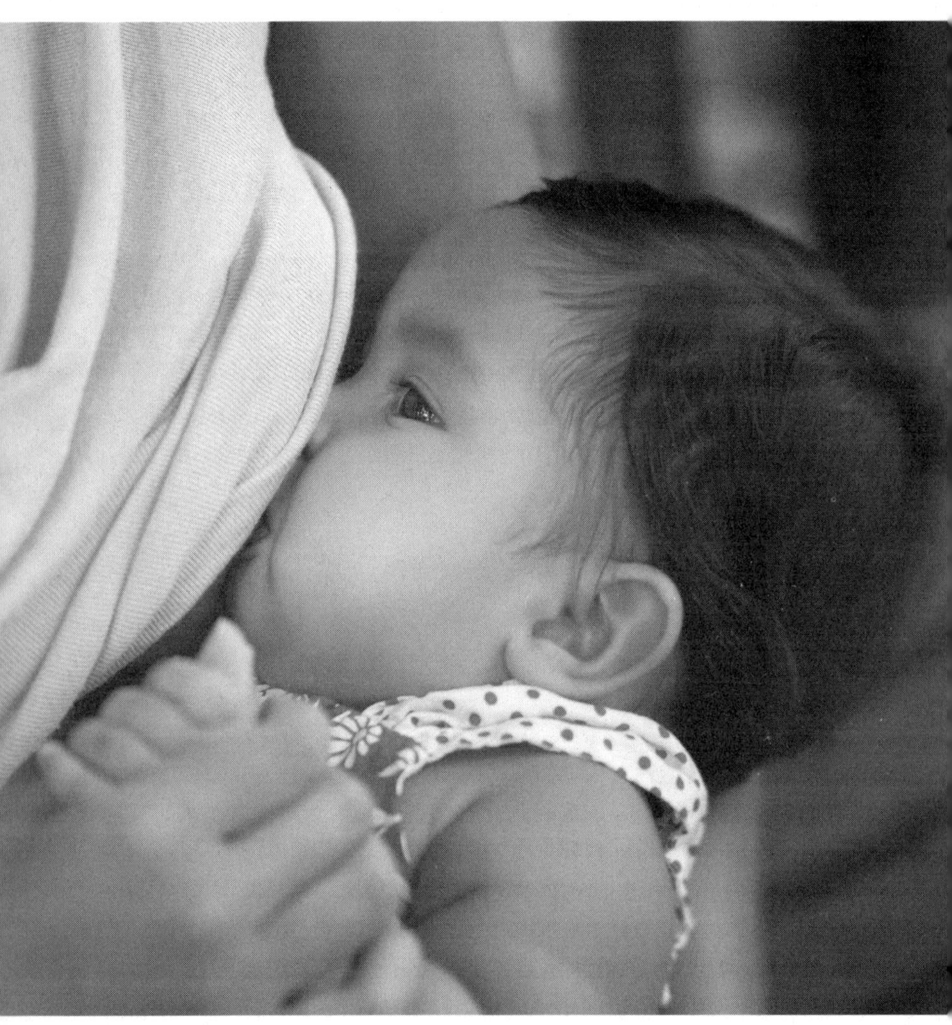

breastfeeding. Skin around nipple (areola) starts darkening due to hormonal changes.

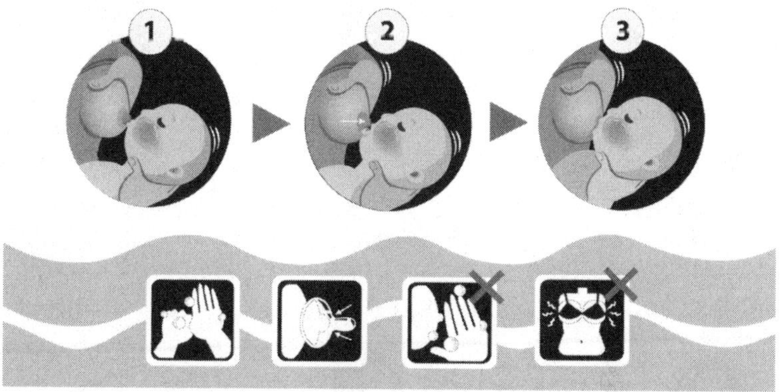

During the last 8 weeks of pregnancy, a pregnant woman should do gentle massage of her breasts while bathing and clean the nipples. Crust may form on or around the nipples due to slight oozing of milk or colostrums (yellowish discharge from nipple) which is more common during the last 2 months of pregnancy. Breasts should be cleaned to remove this crust. Nipples should be kept soft by applying lanolin-based cream on them.

Check your breast during pregnancy

The shape or size of breast has to do nothing with breastfeeding. Asymmetry in breast size or large or big breast is not an obstacle for breastfeeding.

A nipple is a more important structure to breastfeed a baby. When baby sucks on a nipple, it touches the baby's upper jaw (palate) and increases the sucking reflex. So, baby tries to suck more and more. A nipple may be flat, inverted or normal (i.e. everted).

Flat nipples generally come out normally during pregnancy and become normal with baby's sucking.

Breastfeeding Positions

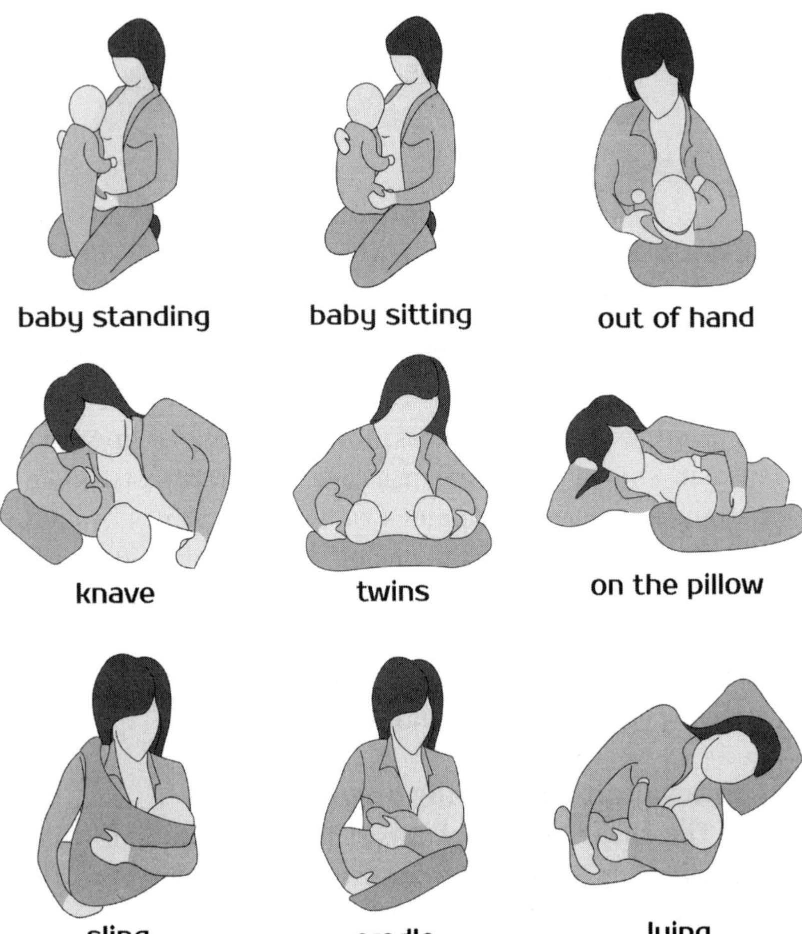

Approximately, 10% mothers have inverted nipples. During breastfeeding, baby sucks on the areola with nipples which may help the nipple to come out but the elasticity of muscles is less in such nipples. So, it should be taken care of during pregnancy.

Care of inverted nipples during pregnancy

Manual: Press the areola towards chest with index and middle finger and try to pull nipples out 5 times. Do this 3 times a day. Start at least in last 6 weeks of pregnancy. Use some lubricant like edible oil or moisturiser to avoid dryness of nipple.

Care of breast during pregnancy

Dos: For few a minutes, keep the nipples daily exposed to the air by avoiding wearing brassieres.

Keep breasts clean and moist.

Donts: Use of soap should be avoided on nipples and areola.

Repeated irritation of nipples by touching it or massaging it may lead to secretion of hormone called oxytocin which in turn leads to preterm labour pains.

Advantages of breastfeeding

There are lots of advantages of breastfeeding.

- The best thing of breast milk is that it is a perfect combination of nature that contains all essential nutrients that the infant needs. There is no need to worry about infection or temperature or freshness and the likes.
- It helps the infant fight against infections and diseases like ear infections, meningitis, diarrhoea

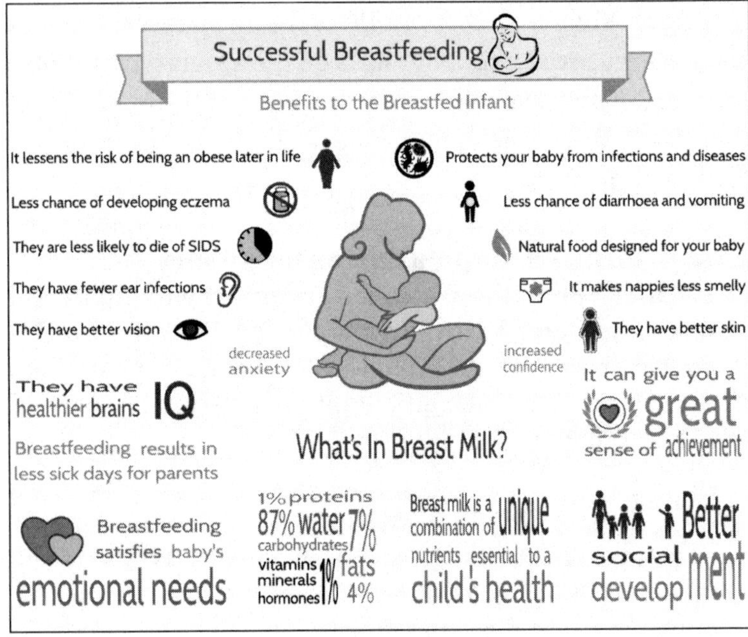
Successful Breastfeeding
Benefits to the Breastfed Infant
It lessens the risk of being an obese later in life
Protects your baby from infections and diseases
Less chance of developing eczema
Less chance of diarrhoea and vomiting
They are less likely to die of SIDS
Natural food designed for your baby
They have fewer ear infections
It makes nappies less smelly
They have better vision
They have better skin
decreased anxiety
increased confidence
They have healthier brains IQ
It can give you a great sense of achievement
Breastfeeding results in less sick days for parents
What's In Breast Milk?
Breastfeeding satisfies baby's emotional needs
1% proteins
87% water
7% carbohydrates
vitamins minerals hormones 1%
fats 4%
Breast milk is a unique combination of nutrients essential to a child's health
Better social development

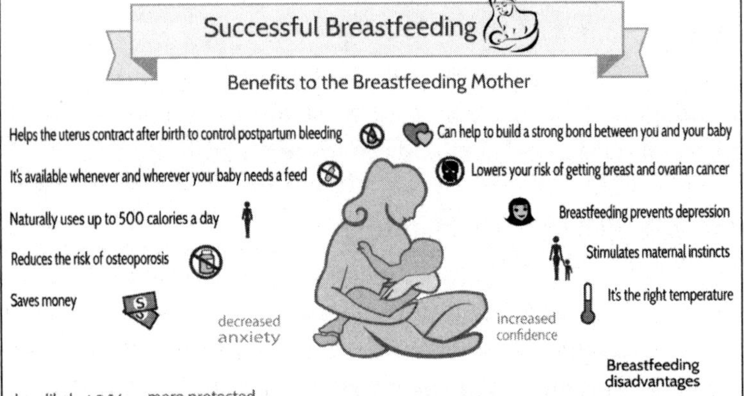
Successful Breastfeeding
Benefits to the Breastfeeding Mother
Helps the uterus contract after birth to control postpartum bleeding
Can help to build a strong bond between you and your baby
It's available whenever and wherever your baby needs a feed
Lowers your risk of getting breast and ovarian cancer
Naturally uses up to 500 calories a day
Breastfeeding prevents depression
Reduces the risk of osteoporosis
Stimulates maternal instincts
Saves money
It's the right temperature
decreased anxiety
increased confidence

less likely to develop 10% cardiovascular diseases
more protected from rheumatoid 50% arthritis
26% less likely to develop diabetes
11% less likely to develop hypertension
What's In Breast Milk?
1% proteins
87% water
7% carbohydrates
vitamins minerals hormones 1%
fats 4%
Breast milk is a unique combination of nutrients essential to a child's health
Breastfeeding disadvantages
Passing on infections
Lack of freedom
Feeding in public restrictions
diet
No one else can feed the baby
It is more difficult for breastfeeding mothers to return to work

and respiratory infection. It is a boon for premature babies and acts as a protective shield against allergies, asthma and obesity.

- Easily accepted and tolerated by infants due to a perfect combination of protein, lactose and fat.
- Breast milk is best for an infant due to its nutritional profile in the form of calories, vitamins and minerals. The same perfect proportion cannot be replicated in commercial mixtures.
- This is a natural source of food for a baby without paying a price for it.
- The infant is exposed to so many food tastes through mother's milk that they develop a broad spectrum of taste preferences and that is how children grow up to eat a variety of food.
- Breastfed infants are less prone to childhood obesity than others.
- Breastfed infants have a higher IQ than those who are not.
- Breastfeeding is helpful to mothers also. Mothers burn calories while breastfeeding and this helps in weight reduction. It also helps in shrinking the uterus post-delivery and lowers the risk of breast, uterine and ovarian cancer.
- There is less chance of pregnancy during lactation.
- Due to breastfeeding, there a special bond is established between the infant and mom. This gives psychological security to the baby.
- Breast milk contains more amount of iron, vitamin D, vitamin C and vitamin E than other type of milk.

Myths of breastfeeding

Myth: Initial breast secretion (colostrums) should be discarded as infant cannot digest it.

Fact: Colostrums are highest-quality protective food for a baby which increases immunity of baby and is easily digestible by a baby.

Myth: Mother having small breasts cannot breastfeed her baby.

Fact: Hormonal changes during pregnancy lead to development of the breast ductules for milk secretion and increase in size of breast which is enough for breastfeeding. So mother with small breasts can lactate enough to breastfeed a baby.

Myth: Mother who has delivered a baby by caesarean section will not be able to feed her baby for a first few days.

Fact: Process of production of breast milk starts during pregnancy (after six months) only. So, it is not related. Even if a mother cannot take food for one day, post-operation, she can still breastfeed immediately. Even a small quantity of milk is useful to the baby.

What is Kangaroo Mother Care (KMC)?

Kangaroo Mother Care is a method of holding a baby that involves skin-to-skin contact with his mother, father or substitute caregiver. The baby, who is naked except for a diaper and piece of cloth covering his/her back, is placed in an upright position against a parent's bare chest.

What is the timing for KMC?

It should be done immediately after birth and as much as you can during first few days of life.

What are the benefits of KMC?

For parents:

It promotes attachment and bonding, improves parental confidence, and helps promote increased milk production and breastfeeding.

For infants (preterm/full term):

It helps in adjusting outside the womb. Preterm infants who experience KMC have improved cognitive development, decreased stress level, reduced pain responses, normalised growth, and positive effects on motor development. It also helps in improvement of sleep pattern of the baby.

□

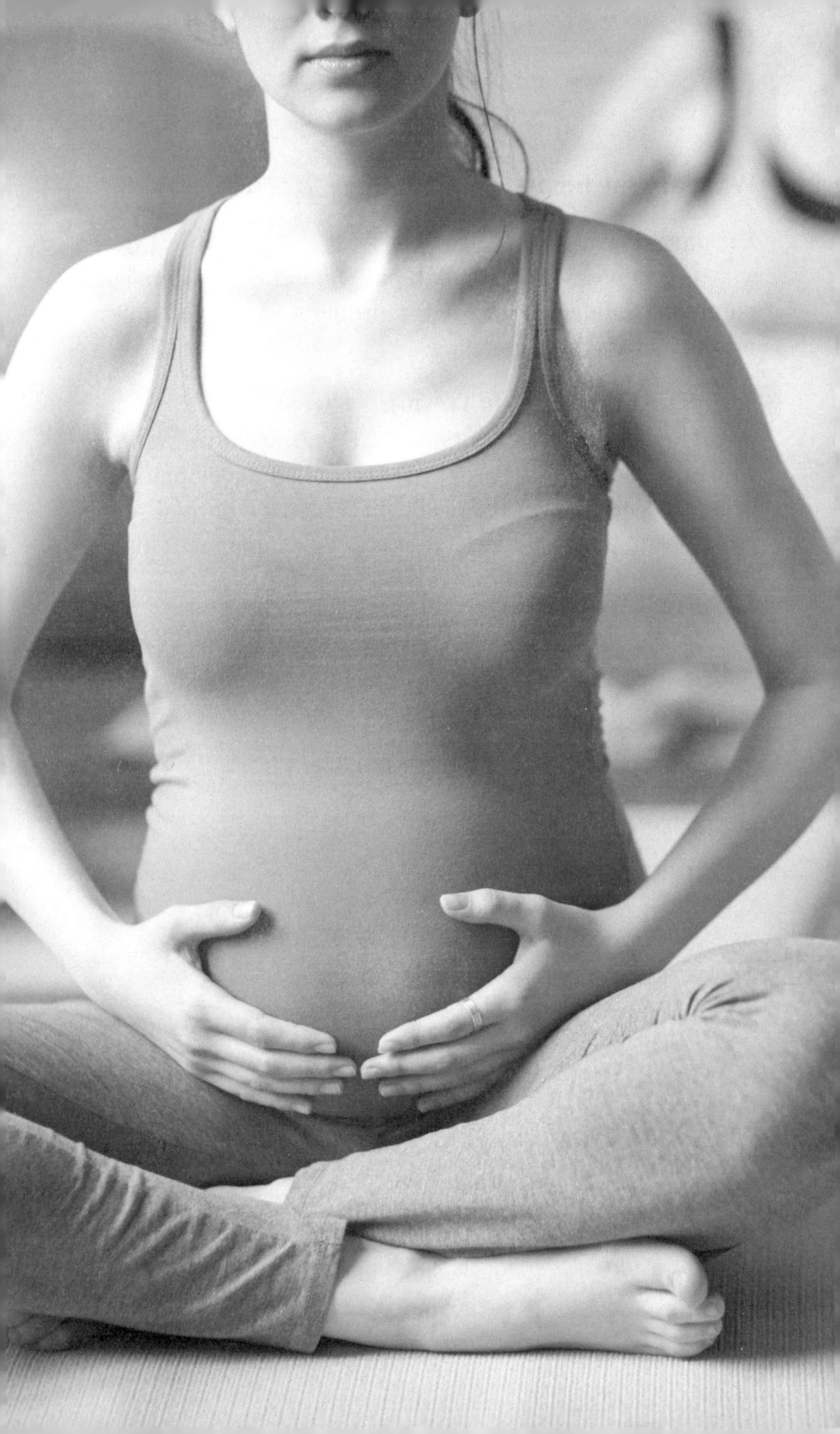

15

Exercises in Pregnancy

During pregnancy, the body experiences dramatic physiological changes that require a carefully designed exercise program. You should know what exercise you can do and what you cannot do.

Why should you exercise?

Most women benefit from exercise throughout pregnancy.

1. Exercise makes you feel better by releasing the hormone endorphin.
2. Helps you sleep better by relieving the stress and anxiety that might make you restless at night.
3. Prepare you and your baby for birth.
4. Regain pre-pregnancy body quickly.

Which exercise should you try?

Always discuss your exercise plan with your doctor.

- Walking is a good exercise. But avoid walking in hot weather.
- *Pranayam*, yoga and breathing exercises are always beneficial and will prepare you for labour.
- Swimming is beneficial.
- Aerobics up to a certain limit.

Avoid

- Weights
- Horse-riding
- Skiing
- Accidental fall
- Excessive jerks

When should a lady limit her exercise?

She may have:

- Early contraction
- Vaginal bleeding
- Pregnancy-induced high BP
- Premature rupture of membrane

Pranayam

Pranayam is also known as 'yogic breathing' or 'controlled deep breathing'.

During pregnancy, you are the sole provider for your baby. Apart from your health, nutrition and fitness, it is important to take care of your breathing pattern as well. *Pranayam* is a technique which teaches you to breathe correctly. It helps you achieve the correct balance of inhaled oxygen and exhaled carbon dioxide –making your lungs stronger and blood purer. This helps your body function properly so that you can take good care of yourself as well as your baby.

Is it safe to practise *Pranayam* during pregnancy

One of the first things you learn in a yoga class is how to breathe fully. There are many techniques for *Pranayam* and though most are considered safe, do ensure you practise under the guidance of a trained instructor.

- A few *Pranayam* techniques may not be suitable during pregnancy – especially where you need to hold your breath for a very long time or take deep forceful breaths that contract your stomach.
- If you suffer from asthma, heart disease or shortness of breath or any other complication, you will need to check with your doctor before you begin *Pranayam*.
- Each technique of *Pranayam* involves a specific breathing ratio and duration of inhalation and exhalation. These will vary for beginners and advanced practitioners. Do ensure you discuss this with your instructor and be honest about what you can do. Listen to your body and slow down if you cannot go up to the next level.
- Avoid following *Pranayam* instructions given through books, television shows and CDs during pregnancy. Your case may be special and only a trained yoga teacher can guide you properly. Also, if done incorrectly, you may end up doing yourself more harm than good.

What are the benefits of *Pranayam*?

When done correctly *Pranayam* offers a lots of benefits:

- *Pranayam* helps to optimise the flow of oxygen that is supplied to your body and your growing baby.
- It helps in the circulation of blood and oxygen which are essential for growing body and for your baby's development.
- It relaxes the mind and helps reduce stress. *Pranayam* is also believed to promote positive

emotional health and self-control. This helps you deal with mood swings, anger and frustration in a much more positive manner.

- It also helps the basic functioning of your body, allowing your body to remove toxins and waste effectively.
- The controlled breathing can be beneficial during labour and childbirth. Learning how to do breathing primes you for labour and childbirth, because it trains you to stay calm when you need it most. When you're afraid during labour, for example, the body produces adrenaline and shuts down the production of oxytocin, a hormone that helps labour progress. Yoga training will help you fight the urge to tighten up when you feel the pain, and show you how to relax and open up instead.

Domestic work

Women can continue with domestic work during pregnancy as it is a good form of exercise. Be careful while walking during pregnancy, avoid falls.

- You intend to burn 150-300 kcal/day.
- Walking for 1 km burns approximately 60-80 kcal, though it is dependent on weight.
- Speed is relatively unimportant in terms of caloric expenditure.

Other exercises in pregnancy

A variety of exercises like cycling, swimming and low impact aerobics are safe in pregnancy.

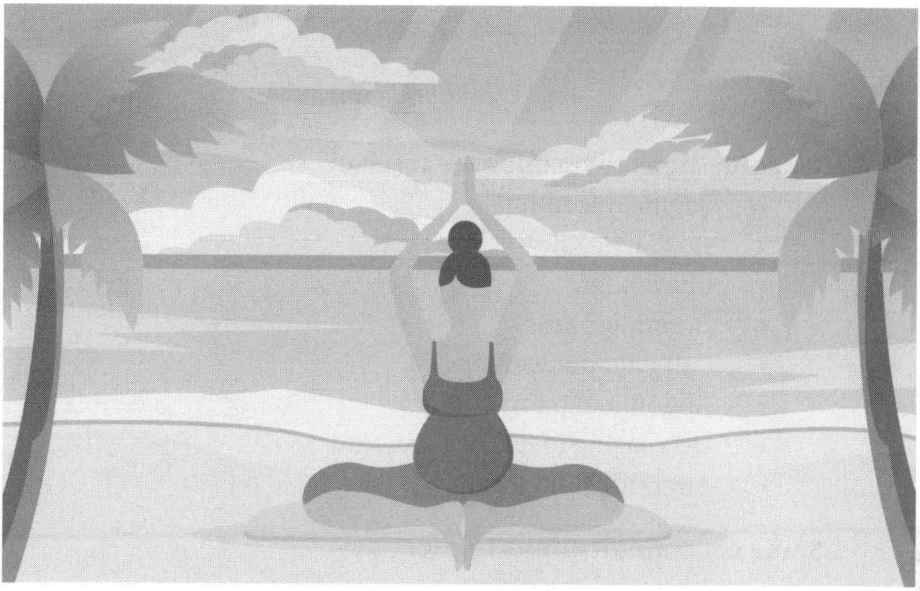

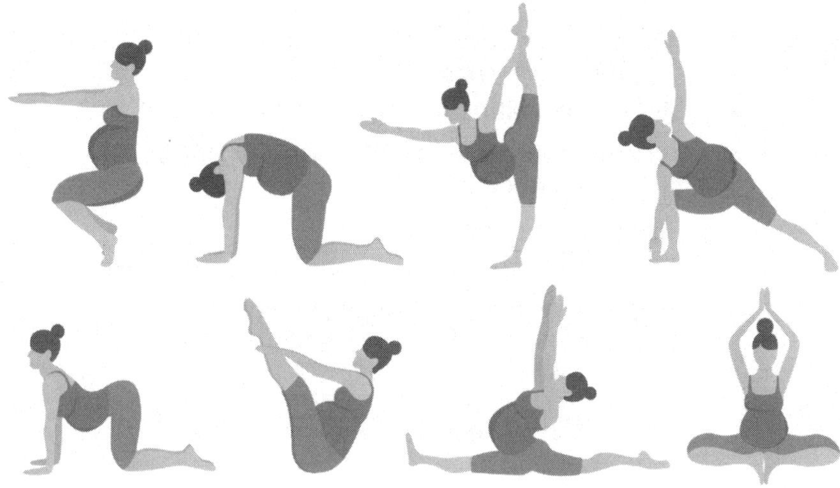

The rule is that whenever you feel exhausted, dizzy or have palpitation stop exercising

Warning signs to terminate exercise:

- Vaginal bleeding
- Headache, dizziness
- Chest pain
- Breathlessness
- Calf pain or swelling
- Abdominal pain
- Decreasing foetal movement
- Amniotic fluid leakage

Some contraindications to exercise:

- Heart or lung disease
- Incompetent cervix or encirclage (stitching of Cervix)
- Multiple gestation at risk of preterm labour
- Persistent 2nd and 3rd trimester bleeding
- Placenta previa
- Ruptured membranes
- Pregnancy-induced hypertension/pre-eclampsia
- Foetal growth restriction in current pregnancy.

□

16

Medicines in Pregnancy

If you are pregnant, you may be wondering whether to take over the counter, medications. Some medicines are safe to take during pregnancy. But others are not or their effects on your baby may not be known. Tell your doctor if you are taking any alternative medicines or supplements.

Safe Medicine

Prenatal vitamins are safe and are important for the growth of the baby.

Some of the common medicines which are safe:

- Allergy: levocetrizine/cetrizine
- Fever: paracetamol/acetaminophen
- Abdominal pain: buscopan, drotin, cyclopam etc.

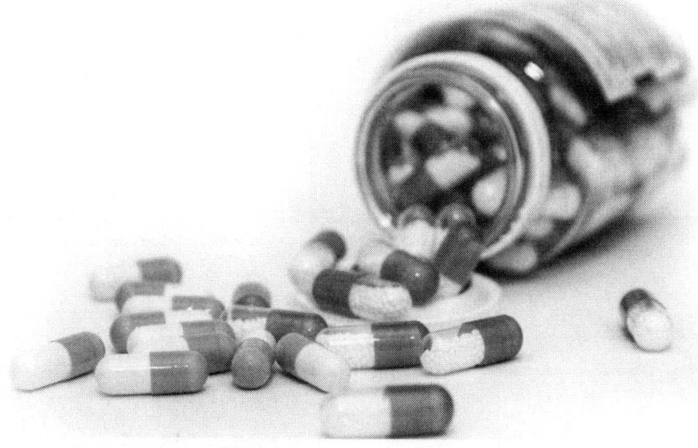

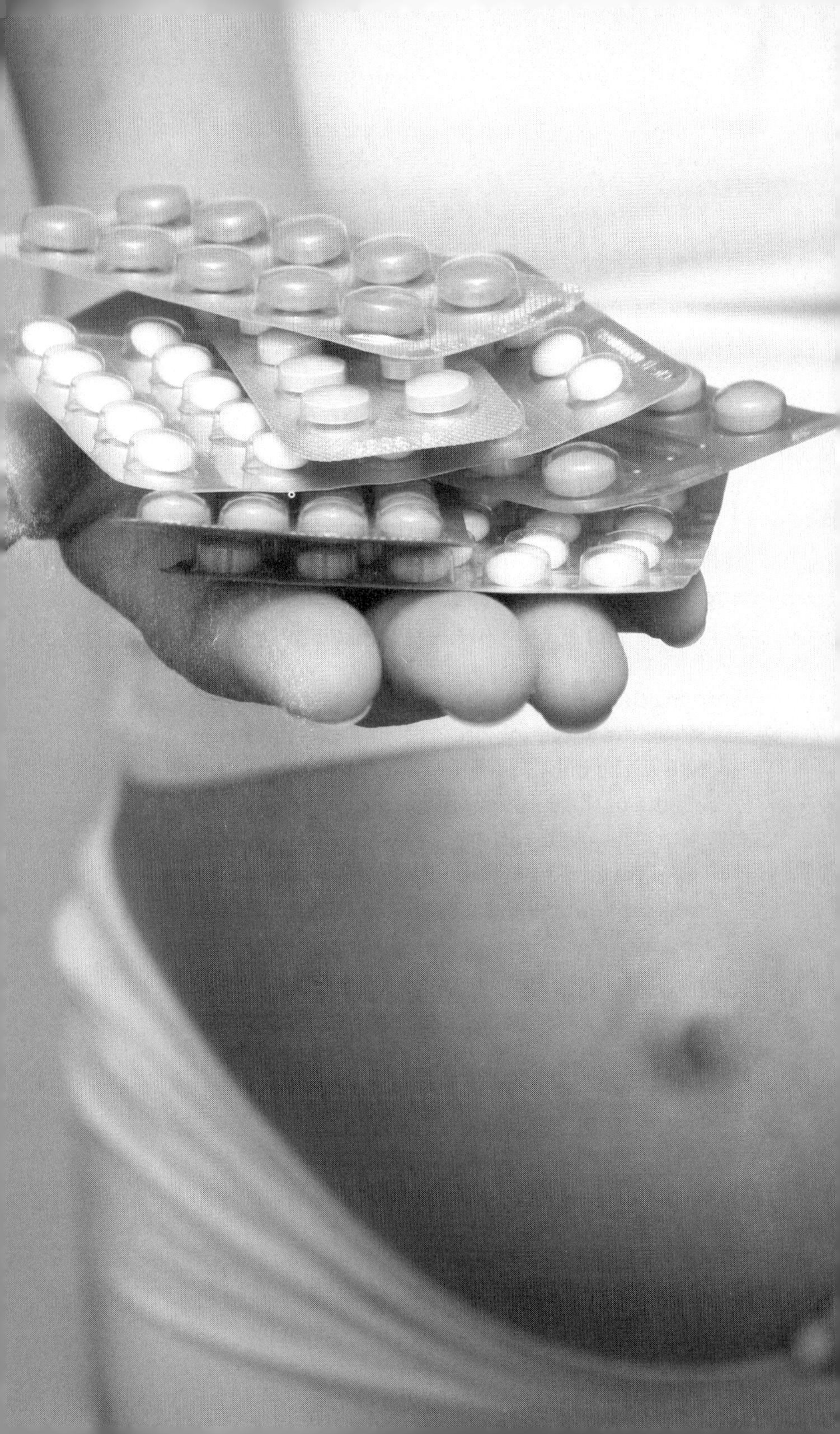

- When during pregnancy, was the medication taken?
- Other health conditions a woman might have.
- Some pregnant women have pre-existing medical conditions like asthma, diabetes, epilepsy, high blood pressure and depression. They may be taking medicines for the same. They have to discuss with their doctor the safest medication suited to them.
- For example, if a diabetic lady on oral hypoglycemic gets pregnant, she may have to switch over to insulin or oral anti diabetic drug safe in pregnancy.
- Females with epilepsy should switch over to the safest medications; otherwise birth defect may occur in baby.
- If you have pre-existing hypertension, anti-hypertensive like Enalapril has to be switched over to safer option like Alphadopa or Nifedipine or Labetalol.
- Sleeping pills, pain-killers should be avoided specially in later months of pregnancy because common analgesics in larger dose over a larger time can decrease fluid inside the amniotic cavity.

The best way is to avoid over-the-counter medications and follow the advice of your doctor.

□

17

Preparing for a Newborn Baby

1. For bath

- Baby bath tub with adjustable sling, backrest/seat.
- Plenty of hooded towels, soft washed clothes.
- Moisturising baby bath soap/shampoo/massage oil/ Moisturising lotion.

2. Bed

- Wash-proof mats.
- Crib sheet, mattress pads.
- Sleeping bag with arm holes.
- Stroller.

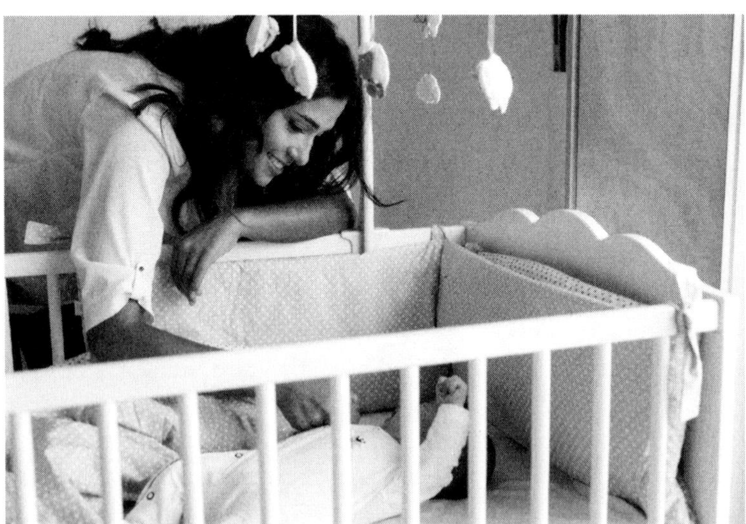

- Crib.
- Car seat if you are driving alone with your baby.

3. For entertainment

- Brightly coloured, high-contrast or soft musical toys.
- Swing.

4. Diapers

- Nappies.
- Diaper-cloths/disposable.
- Wipes.
- Diaper-rash cream.
- Dettol antiseptic solution to clean baby's clothes and nappies.
- Cotton-wool pads to clean baby.
- Plastic bags for soiled diapers.

5. Common medicines

- Saline nasal drops for stuffy nose.
- Bulb or syringe for cleaning nose.
- Thermometer.
- Nail clipper.
- Nail filer.

6. Cotton clothes

□

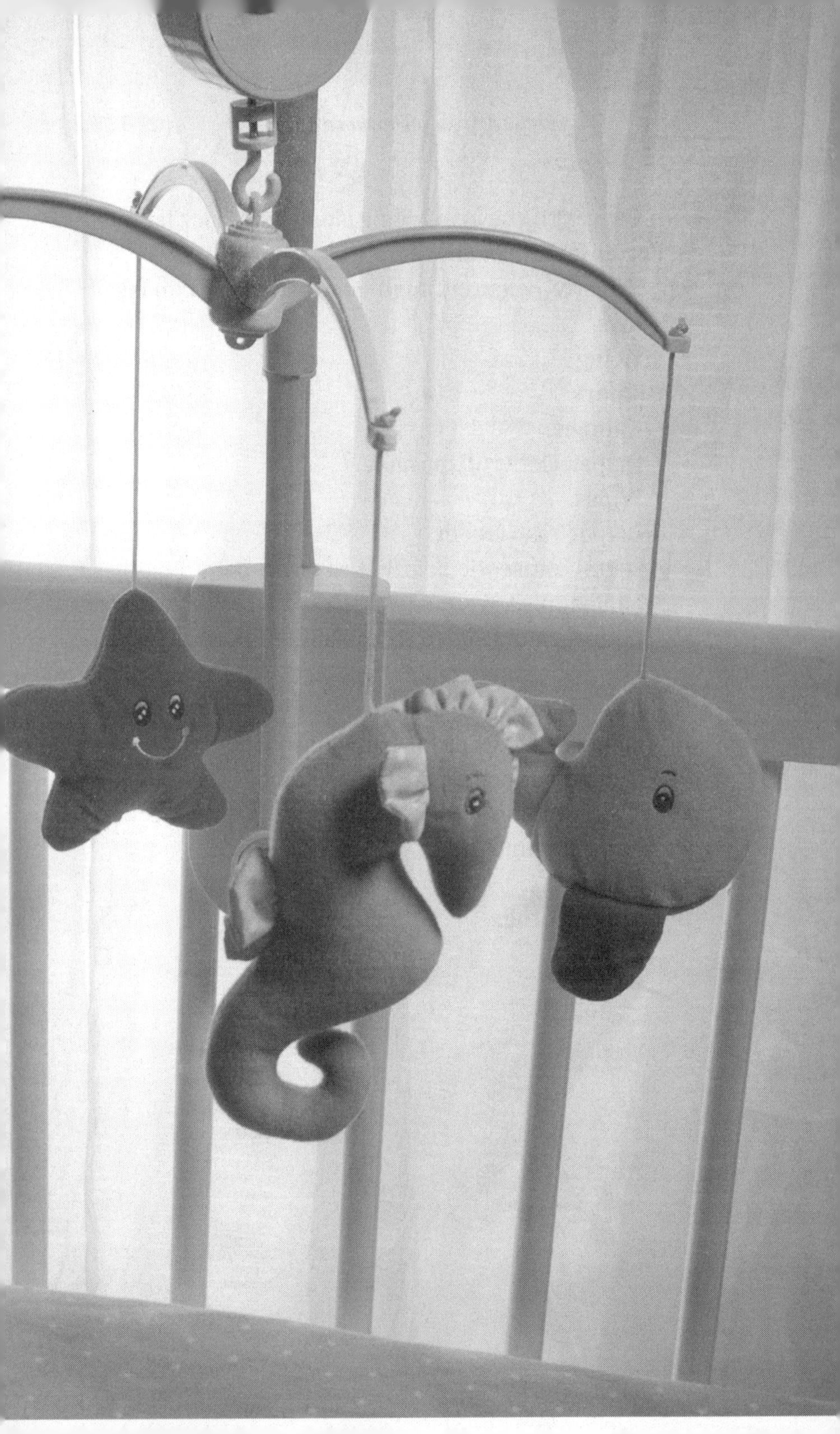

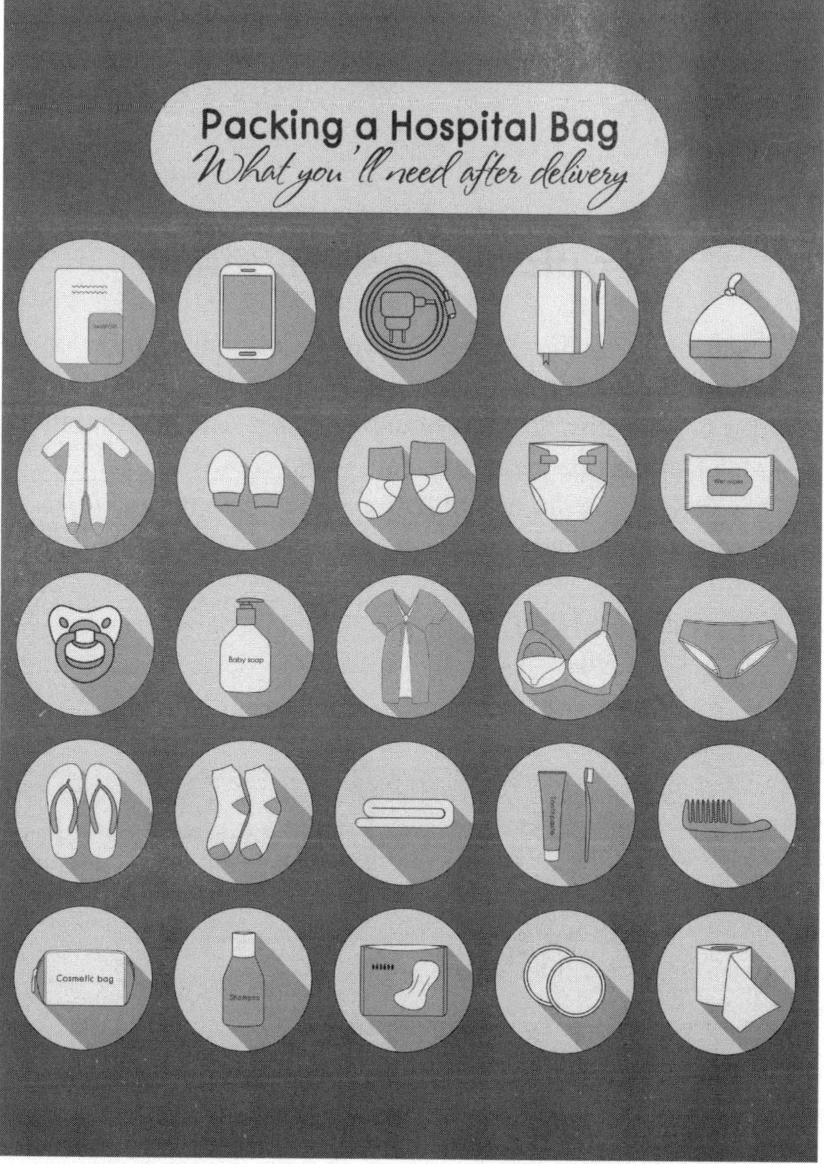
Packing a Hospital Bag
What you'll need after delivery
Baby soap
Toothpaste
Cosmetic bag
Shampoo

18

Checklist for Hospitalisation

During pregnancy, there is always a small chance for preterm delivery or premature delivery at any time after 6-7 months. So, you should keep bag ready so that in case of an emergency, you remain stress-free.

You can prepare two bags: One for labour and you, other for you after delivery and for baby.

For labour and you

1. Your file
2. Towel

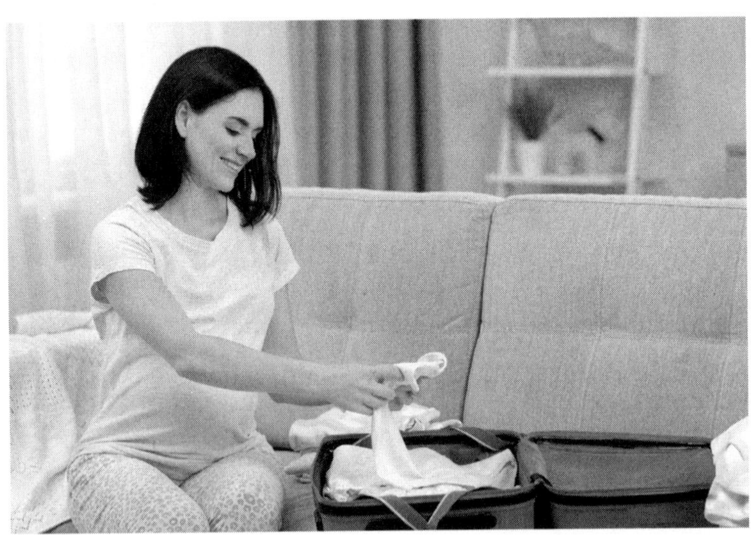

3. One *pyjama* or night-suit with front opening
4. Two packs of maternity pads.
5. Clothes and socks
6. Breast pads
7. Toiletries: hairband, hairbrush, lipbalm, soaps/ face-wash, toothpaste, etc.
8. High energy snacks and juices
9. Baby body suit and caps
10. Camera
11. Slippers
12. Books, magazine, music etc. to relax
13. Disposable panties

Post-birth/baby

1. *Pyjamas*/night gown with front openings
2. Nursing bras
3. Cotton, wool pads
4. Mirrors, disposable tissues
5. Nappies and nappy sacs/bags
6. Nappy rash cream
7. Socks/booties
8. Baby brush/shampoo
9. Blankets
10. Earplugs
11. Baby wipes, non-perfumed

□

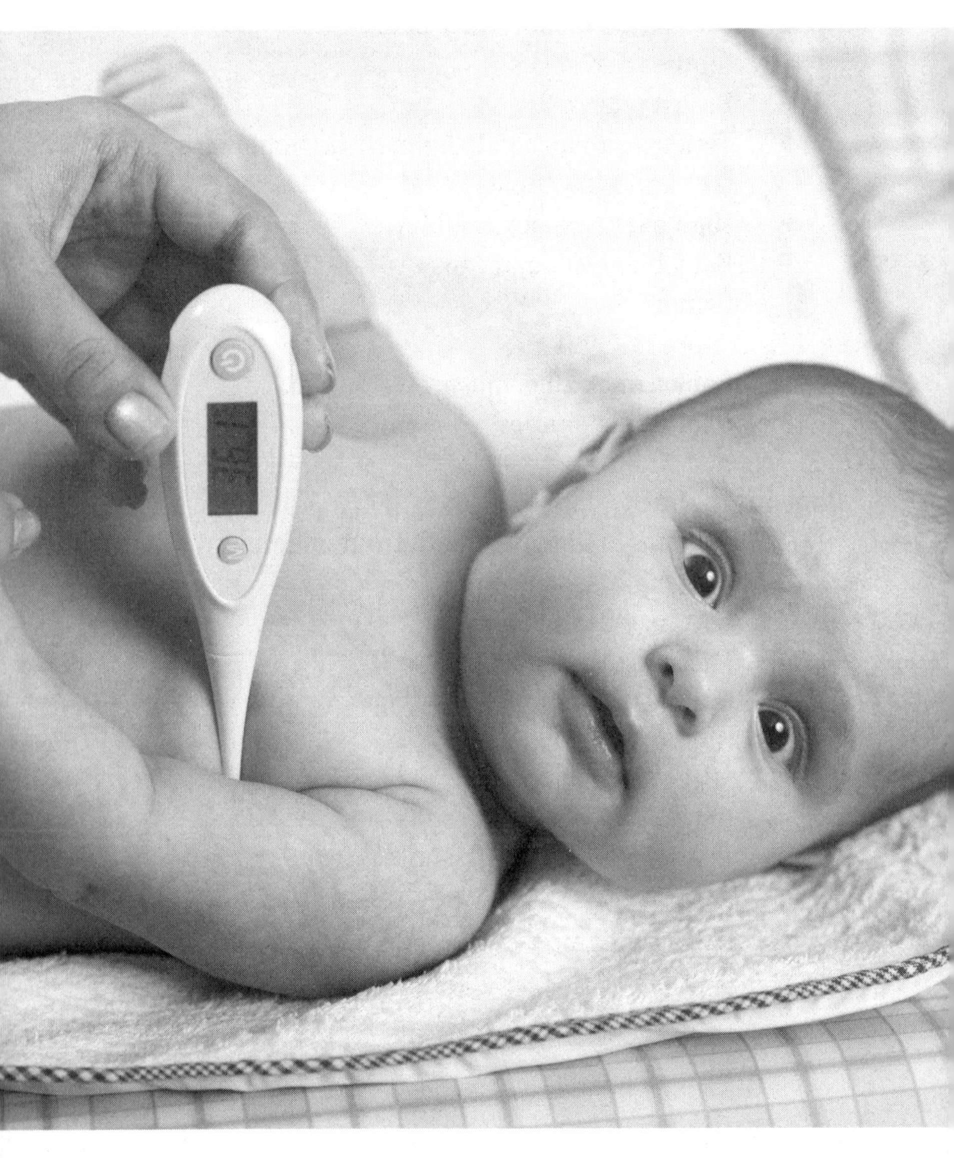

19

Warning Signs in Newborns

The warning signs in which you should contact a doctor immediately are as follows:

1. If your baby doesn't pass a greenish black stool (Meconium) within 36-48 hours of birth.
2. If your baby doesn't pass urine within 24 hours of birth or failure to urinate every 6-8 hours or fewer than 5 wet diapers in 24 hours.
3. *Jaundice*: Whites of eyes are turning yellow, skin below nipple line turning yellow.
4. *Umbilical cord problem*: Redness around the cord, foul odour or pus, bright red-coloured bleeding that makes a quarter-sized spot on the diaper or T-shirt.
5. *Vomiting*: If it is forceful or more frequent than usual (more than spitting up).
6. *Feeding problems*: Repeatedly refuses feeding for more than 6-8 hours.
7. Excessively or uncharacteristically fussy or irritable, unusually lethargic or sleepy.
8. Fever more than 100ºF.
9. *Dehydration*: If you pinch the baby's skin, it stays pinched up, wrinkled, crepe paper-like with dry mouth, dark yellow urine and sunken fontanelle.

10. *Diarrhoea*: Frequent and watery stool causing weight loss with blood or mucus in stool.
11. *Breathing problems*: Signs like blue lips, struggling for breath, flaring of nostrils, and deep indentation of the chest when breathing.
12. *Cyanosis*: Bluish colour of skin, nails.
13. *Floppy muscle tone*: Unequal limb movements on both sides or restriction of movements of any joint or limb.
14. White patches on the tongue or inside the mouth.
15. Bright red bleeding, swelling, foul-smelling discharge during urination.
16. *Redness of eyes*: Most common in summer.
17. *Bowel movement*: Constipation with forceful vomiting and distension of abdomen.
18. Hiccups, sneezing and yawning: Hiccup usually occurs after feeding due to distension of stomach and irritation of diaphragm.

    Sneezing is due to irritation of nostrils by secretions and it is normal.

    Yawning is also normal.
19. *Excessive crying*: It is usually due to hunger or some discomfort like wetness of diaper or evacuation of hard stool or before passing urine or diaper rash.
20. *Evening colic*: Excessive crying with flushed face occurs at a precise time everyday and for that, you can take your baby for a drive, cuddle, kiss or keep him in a prone position.

□

20

Pregnancy and Working Women

You may be able to continue working until the day you deliver or close to it, if you are healthy and have a normal pregnancy. You may tire more easily towards the end of your pregnancy. So, take it as easily as possible.

Factors at workplace that lead to low birthweight babies and high blood pressure in pregnancy and chance of premature delivery are follow:

- Physically strenuous activities including lifting heavy weights.
- Standing for long periods.
- Irregular and excessive hours.

If you have a strenuous job, you can try switching to a less physically taxing type of work like a desk job if possible or take occasional leave to relieve fatigue.

If you work in a field where you come into contact with known reproductive hazards, such as heavy metals like lead and mercury, chemicals, such as organic solvents, certain biological agents, and radiation, you will need to change your job or take leave from work. These are teratogens – agents that can cause problems like miscarriage, preterm delivery, structural birth defects and abnormal foetal and infant development when a woman is exposed to them during or even prior to pregnancy.

You're likely to come into contact with these hazards while working in places, such as computer chip factories, dry-cleaning plants, rubber factories, operating rooms, darkrooms, tollbooths, pottery studios, ship-building plants, and printing presses, etc.

The most common conditions, which might cause you to stop working or decrease your hours during pregnancy, are:

- If you are at risk for preterm labour. This includes women who are expecting twins or more multiples.
- If you have high blood pressure or are at risk for pre-eclampsia.
- If you have a cervical insufficiency or a history of late miscarriage.
- If your baby isn't growing properly.

What care can you take at your workplace?

- Be prepared to reach your hospital if you experience the need to do so.
- Plan your leave and your work and projects.
- Take your seniors and colleagues in confidence and keep them updated of anything unusual.
- Take breaks.

1. If you've been standing, put your feet up or walk around, moving the muscles helps push fluid out of the feet and legs and backup to the heart to be recirculated.
2. If you've been sitting, stand and walk around every two hours. This will help decrease swelling in your feet and ankles, and it should keep you more comfortable.

- Wear comfortable shoes and loose clothing.
- Drink a lot of water. This will also give you a chance to take a break.
- Go to the bathroom as often as you need to.

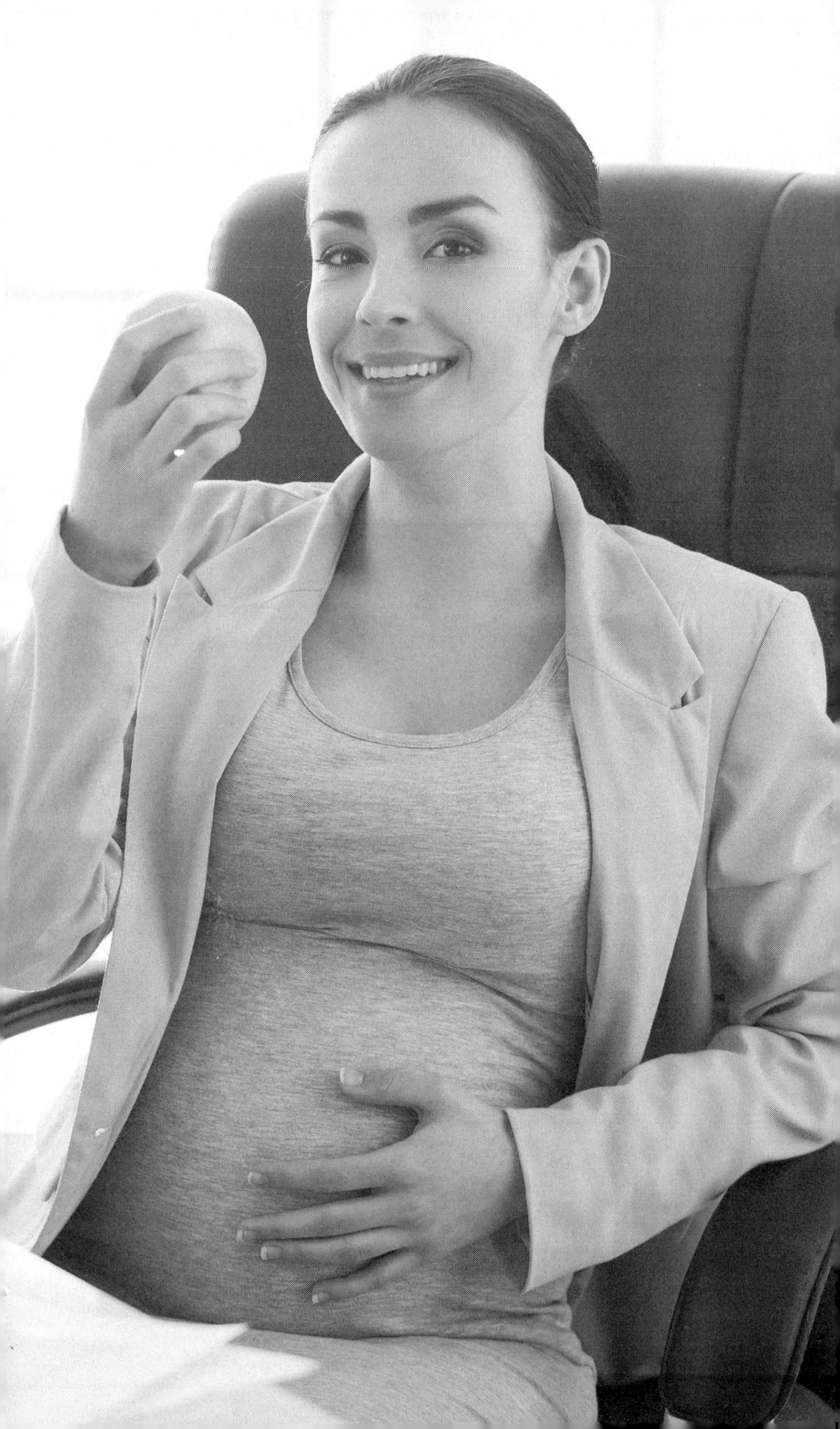

- Take time to eat regular meals and have nutritious snacks. Carry home-cooked healthy food and snacks with you to have frequent snacks and a healthy lunch. Regular snacking helps prevent drops in blood sugar and morning sickness. Choose lunches that are balanced and nutritious whenever you can.
- Reduce stress. If you can't eliminate a stress factor in your workplace, try to find ways to manage it, such as stretching, deep

WORKING DAY A PREGNANT
WOMAN SHOULD NOT EXCEED
SIX HOURS.
WAREHOUSE
DURING PREGNANCY
PROHIBITED THE CARRYING
AND MOVEMENT OF HEAVY
OBJECTS.

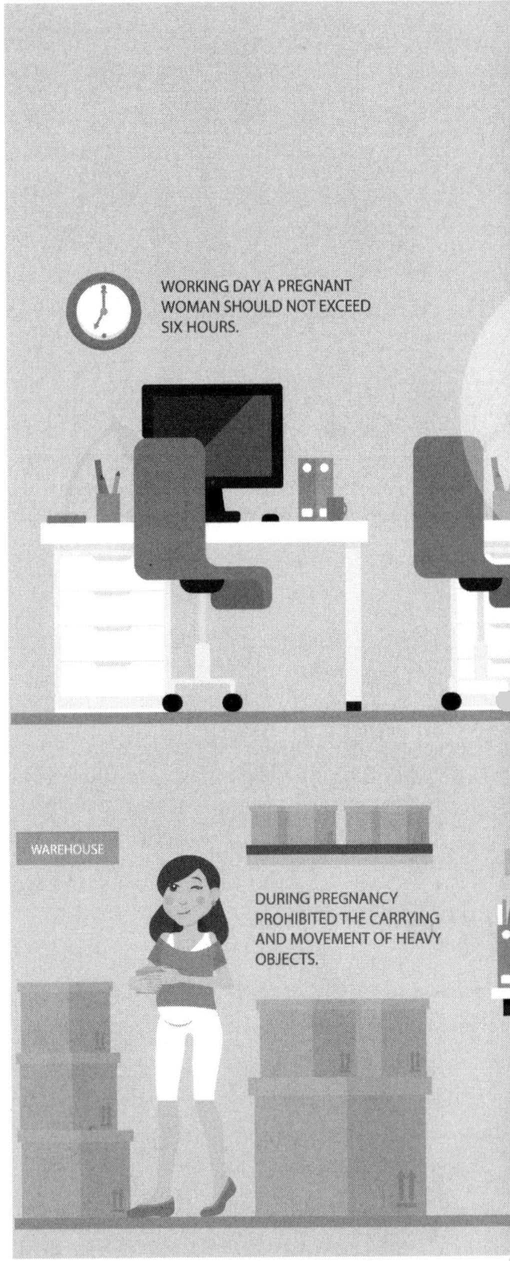

Infographic

WORK DURING PREGNANCY

IN THE CASE OF SEDENTARY WORK, YOU SHOULD REGULARLY TAKE SMALL BREAKS TO WARM UP, WALK.

IT IS DESIRABLE TO ARRANGE SMALL SNACKS — DRIED FRUIT, MUESLI, APPLES, CRACKERS.

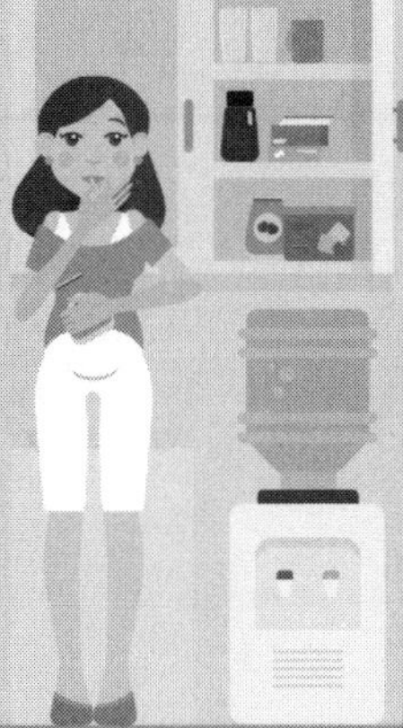

NOT TO OVERWORK AND NOT TO BE NERVOUS.

IT IS NOT RECOMMENDED TO WORK WITH A LONG STANDING (MORE THAN 3 HOURS PER DAY)

IT IS VERY IMPORTANT TO EAT RIGHT. TO TAKE FOOD FROM HOME OR EAT IN THE DINING ROOM.

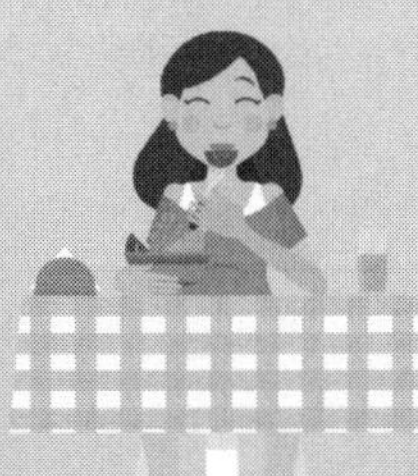

A PREGNANT WOMAN MUST NOT WORK OVERTIME AND WEEKENDS.

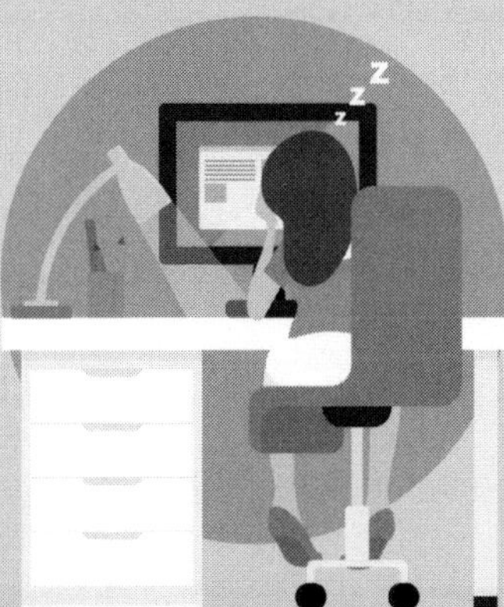

breathing exercises or yoga, or simply taking a short walk.

- Rest when you can. The more strenuous your job is, the more you should reduce physical activity outside of work. If you find yourself feeling fatigued, take an occasional leave to rest.
- Turn down overtime, especially in jobs requiring physical activity.
- Accept help. If your co-workers want to help you a little for your baby and you don't mind, then let them help. Consider yourself lucky to be in a supportive workplace. This is a rare and special time in your life, and it would be a shame to have to pretend that nothing has changed everyday when you're at work.

□

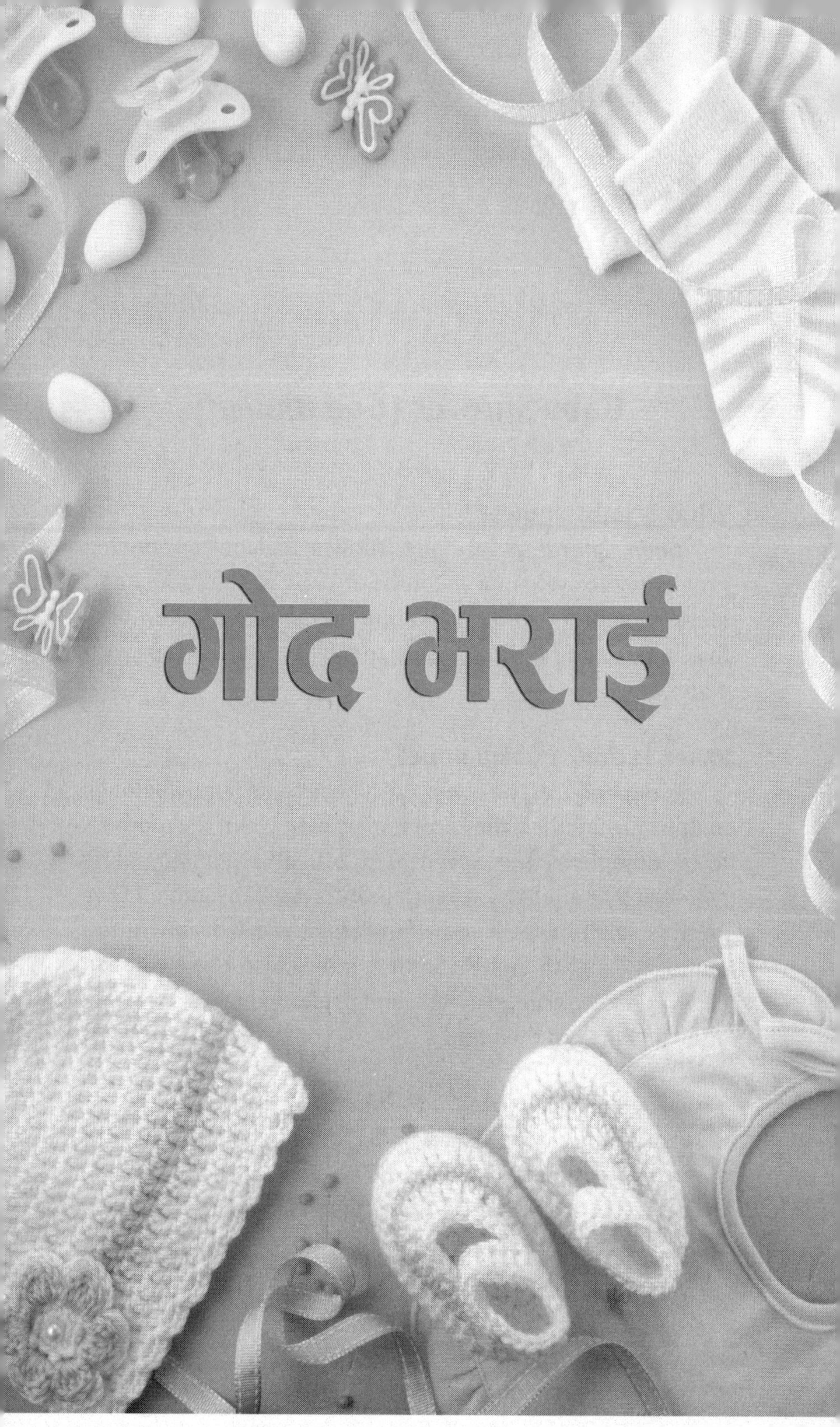

गोद भराई

21

Baby Shower (*God Bharai*)

What is baby shower?

Godh bharai is a baby shower celebrated during pregnancy to welcome the unborn baby to the family and bless the mother-to-be with abundant joys of motherhood. In Hindi, *Godh bharai* literally means to 'fill the lap' with abundance.

When is *Godh bharai* done?

It depends on the community which the family belongs to. In some families, the ceremony is held when the mother-to-be completes her seventh month of pregnancy. It is believed that after the seventh month, the baby and mother are in a safe phase. In some families, it is celebrated at the end of the eighth month. Some families also choose not to have a *Godh bharai* ceremony and prefer to have a puja only after the birth of the baby.

Tips for an enjoyable *Godh bharai*

Your *Godh bharai* is a wonderful time for the family to come together and celebrate your pregnancy and the arrival of your little one. Here are a few tips to help you enjoy your special day.

- It is a good idea to get adequate rest before the ceremony as it may get hectic and tiring for you.
- You may want to select a *saree, lehenga or salwar kameez* for the occasion according to the weather. Heavily embroidered brocades or silks may get uncomfortable during peak summer months.
- The feast prepared for *Godh bharai* is often extensive, including sweets and deep-fried savouries. Try to eat small quantities of what you like and politely refuse extra portions if you feel full.
- If you want to do something to entertain your guests, you can hire a few *mehendi* artists who can apply *henna tattoos* or create *mehendi* designs on the hands of your guests.

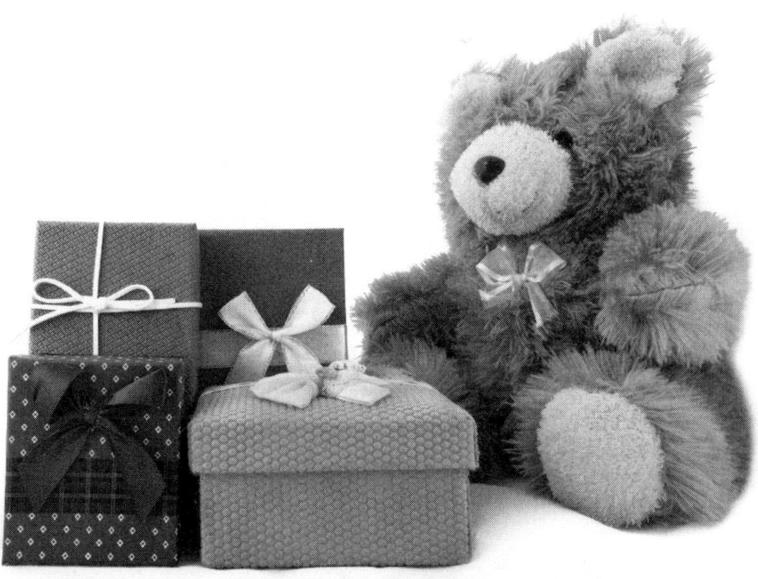

- You may also want to give small tokens of appreciation, such as *dupattas*, stoles, scarves, pretty bangles, cosmetics, perfumes or a set of *kumkum tikkas* as return gifts.

Your *Godh bharai* is a great occasion to meet friends and family. You can build a support group of close friends and relatives who will be there for you and to help you through the last trimester of your pregnancy and when your baby arrives.

□

22
Garbha Sanskar

Garbha Sanskar is all about keeping yourself in a good state emotionally, mentally, physically and spiritually for the sake of your growing baby.

To do this, ancient scriptures suggest:

- Listening to music
- Thinking positive
- Eating healthy
- Yoga
- Meditation and prayer
- Being creative
- Communicating with your unborn child

How does music help my growing baby?

Your unborn baby can hear and respond to sounds from the seventh month onwards. So, if you're listening to music, it's likely that it will be able to hear it too. Some experts believe that listening to music will stimulate your baby's brain development as well as develop its sense of hearing. You could listen to the soothing tunes of instruments like the sitar or the violin. You could also chant pregnancy *shlokas* or sing songs to your baby. Many stores also sell music made especially for pregnant women. Besides stimulating your baby, listening to music can be an excellent stress buster for you.

How do I keep positive throughout my pregnancy?

During pregnancy, unpredictable hormone levels can make you more emotional than usual. So, even though you might want to keep happy and stress-free throughout, you are likely to have ups and downs. You can keep yourself happy by thinking of the things you like doing and trying your best to take time out for them.

If you do not have time for a hobby, even reading books or watching a good movie can do the trick. According to *Garbha sanskar,* it is believed that reading educative books during pregnancy will pass on the wisdom to the child. So, for ages, pregnant women have been encouraged to read mythological stories and scriptures in the hope that good moral values would reach their babies. If you'd prefer something more modern, you could read other books. Whether it's about cooking, self-help, romance, nursery rhymes or fairy tales, read something that makes you feel happy. A good comedy or movie with a happy ending can also lift your spirits.

Give positive suggestions to yourself like

- Nothing will go wrong. Your doctors are very good and will take care of any problems. So, you need not worry.
- You are healthy and capable of handling pregnancy and childbirth.
- Your child is healthy, developing well, etc.
- You could also just simply remember good moments in your life, or go on a holiday. Or perhaps, you could put up photographs of your loved ones around you.

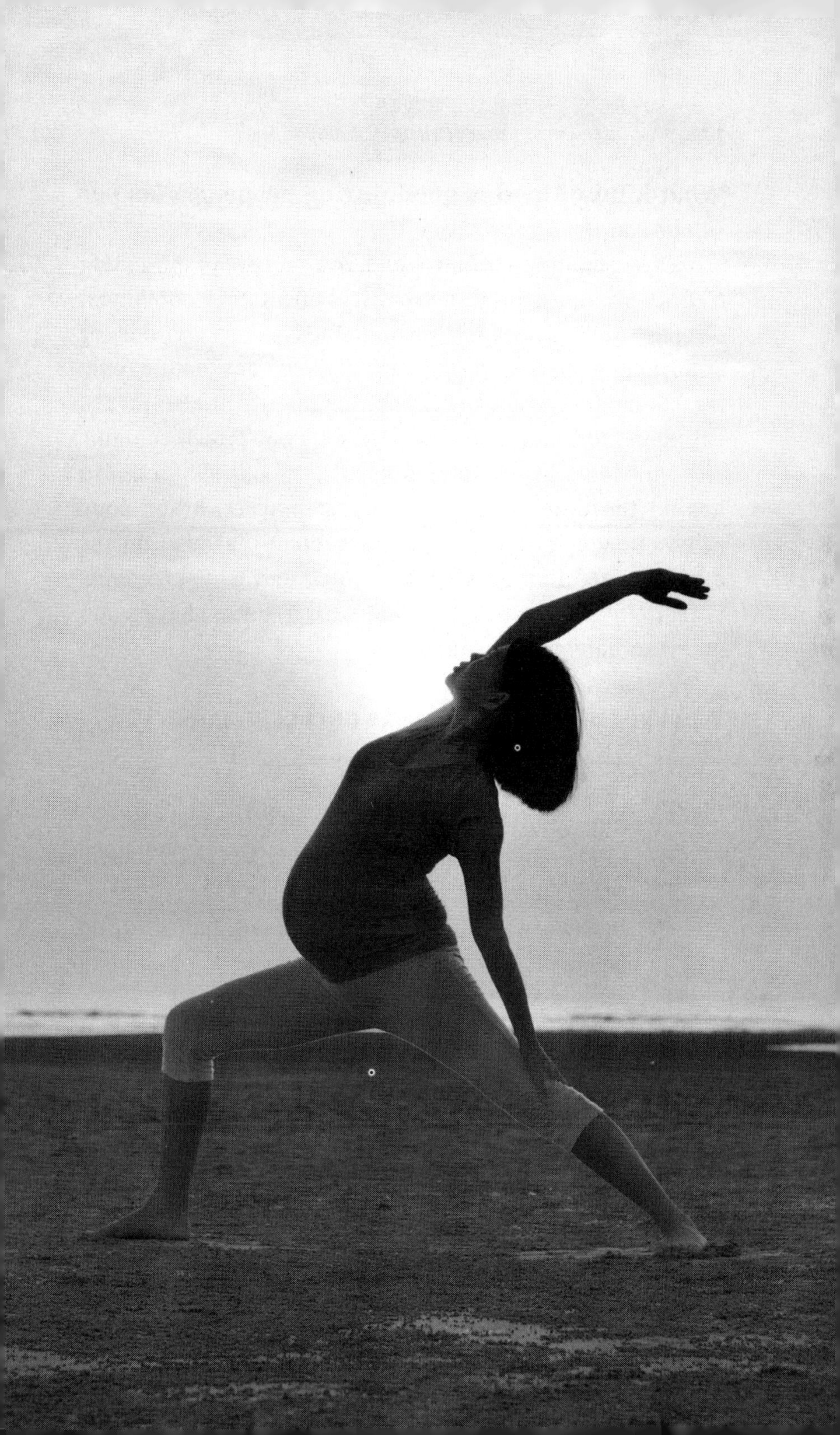

What kind of food is good during pregnancy as per *Garbha sanskar*?

Of everything you do while you are pregnant, eating right is probably the thing that will affect your baby most directly. *Garbha sanskar* recommends a '*saatvik*' diet or a pure diet during pregnancy. This means eating only freshly-made meals using fresh ingredients. It also means eating in moderation. A *saatvik* dish is one which contains vital nutrients in balanced proportions. *Saatvik* food also has all the different kinds of taste – sweet, bitter, sour, salty, pungent and astringent. A *saatvik* diet also means avoiding food that is spicy, fermented and which contains preservatives. It is believed that such a diet will keep you and your baby healthy and pure.

What are the benefits of yoga during pregnancy?

Yoga during pregnancy is said to:

- Increase the flexibility and elasticity of your muscles, which would be useful during labour.
- Improve your blood circulation, which will help reduce pregnancy-related backaches and leg cramps.
- Increase your capacity to bear pain during pregnancy and labour.
- Help in keeping your weight in check.
- Calm and relax you.
- The *pranayam* and breathing techniques employed in yoga are particularly relaxing.

How will meditation and praying help during pregnancy?

Meditation is an integral part of yoga as well as *Garbha sanskar*. It helps give you peace of mind and improve your concentration. In doing so, it is believed that you are helping your baby in the same way. You are helping to develop the ability to stay calm in stressful circumstances.

Meditation involves trying to achieve a 'zero state of mind', which is when you are thinking about nothing, and your mind is blank. While trying to meditate, you can visualise your baby and with each breath, think of all the wonderful experiences you want to share with her. Many mothers find that this process brings them joy and helps them connect better with their growing babies.

Praying and other spiritual activities are an important part of *Garbha sanskar*. It is believed to play a role in the spiritual development of your baby. There are *mantras* and *shlokas* that are specifically recited for the unborn baby. These include prayers to bless the baby with good attributes, like intelligence, good health, happiness and good moral values.

How will creativity help in pregnancy?

Taking up a hobby during pregnancy keeps your mind active, and is believed to enhance your baby's overall development. You can try your hand at various creative pastimes like painting and knitting. Nowadays, many expecting mothers try their hands at maths, classical music, chess or science-based crafts in an effort to enhance their baby's intelligence. If nothing else, a hobby gives you something interesting to do, and is an excellent stress-buster.

How do I communicate with my unborn baby?

Caressing, talking and singing to your tummy are popular ways of communicating. You and your husband could take turns to caress your tummy. You could talk to your baby about a different topic everyday. Tell her how happy you are to have her in your life, share funny anecdotes about the family, or talk about your plans for the future. You may find this bizarre at first. Give it time; it will soon grow on you.

Communicating with your baby, or '*Garbha Samwaad*', is considered to be the most important aspect of *Garbha Sanskar*. It is believed to stimulate senses, and contribute to mental and physical growth. It can also go a long way towards building a strong bond between you and your baby.

Are there any new techniques taught at *Garbha Sanskar* workshops these days?

The concept of *Garbha Sanskar* is becoming increasingly popular. As a result, a number of *Sarbha sanskar* workshops have cropped up to help pregnant mothers understand and practise *Garbha Sanskar*. Some workshops have introduced new techniques based on the same principle of positively enhancing the development of the mother and her baby. Here are some of them:

Autosuggestion and autohypnosis

This is a meditation technique based on the principle that any idea exclusively occupying the mind can turn into reality. So, this technique requires the pregnant mother to make her mind go completely blank, and then start imagining her baby inside is growing well and is healthy. This way you are willing your baby to be healthy, and you will also be creating a positive bond with her.

Colour therapy: This is the use of light and colour to balance your physical, emotional, spiritual or mental energy. It is believed that such therapy can uplift you and consequently, your baby. Some believe that it develops your baby's eyes.

Aromatherapy: This is the use of essential oils and other aromatic substances to soothe the body and mind and sharpen your five senses. Some workshops also provide herbal medicines or supplements. It is best to check with your doctor before you take any of these.

□

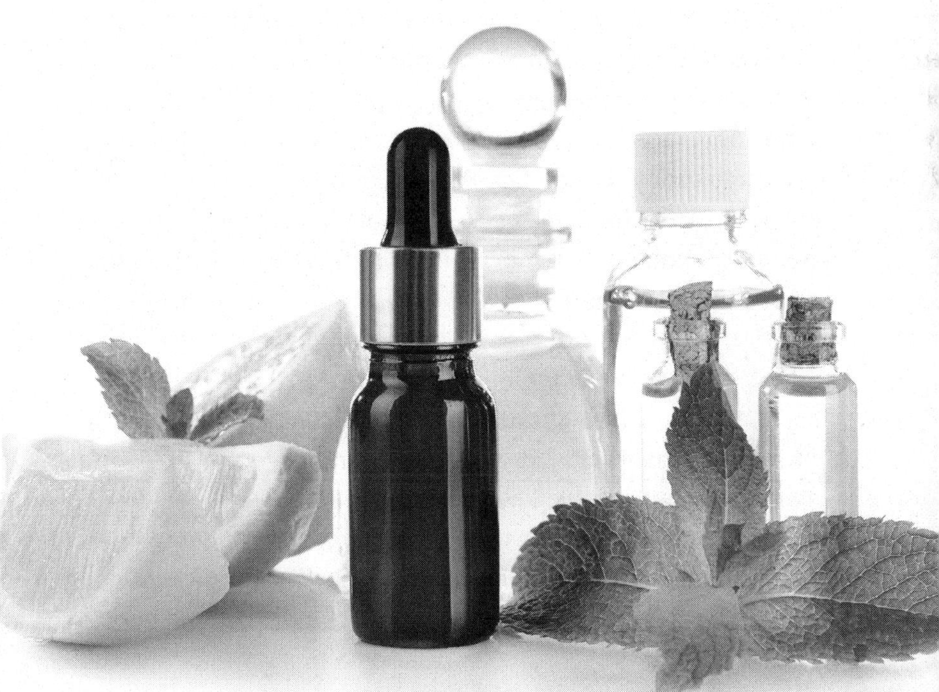

23
Fatherhood

Becoming a father and a parent can be a transformational process for a man too. When a man becomes a father, through loving his child, partner and family, he comes in contact with a deep paternal masculinity. When a child enters a man's life, a new depth of feelings and emotions is awakened within him.

Just because the woman is the one carrying the baby, it doesn't mean that pregnancy has no impact on the father. Whether the pregnancy has been planned for months or years, or is unexpected, you'll probably feel a range of emotions. A baby means new responsibilities, whatever your age that you may not feel ready for.

You and the mother-to-be may have mixed feelings about pregnancy. It's normal for both of you to feel like this. The first pregnancy is a very important event. It will change your life and change can be frightening even if it's something you've been looking forward to.

You can't be pregnant, but you can participate by being an active observer. Let your wife know you're enjoying seeing her belly grow. Feel the baby kick.

Pregnancy is seen as mostly a mom thing. Few women believe that dad really gets it. And the fact is they mostly don't. They talk about it. They show interest. They *empathise* (without going overboard). They even try to read about it, at least a little.

Men today want to participate in the birth process. They want to be there with and for their partners. They want to be involved in offering support and love.

Fathers who are able to participate in the birth of their child often report that the sharing of this experience with their partner/wife remains one of the most important moments in their relationship and in their lives. Even if the birth is difficult or a cesarean delivery, men still feel strongly about being together at this special time. Fathers' importance in participating at the birth is finally getting the acknowledgment it deserves.

Go the extra mile (What to do when you are to become a father?)

- Try to make it to at least some of your wife's many prenatal care appointments, and ask questions. (It shows you're involved, not just a bystander.)
- Also, don't miss the chance to get a glimpse of your baby during an ultrasound.
- If your partner has an amniocentesis or other procedure to test for genetic defects, make sure you're there.
- As your wife tries to modify her diet, and drink more fluids, you can support her by sharing these lifestyle changes. Eliminate "bad-for-baby" foods that might tempt her.
- Take care of your own health also.
- Cut down on or cut out alcohol intake yourself.
- Don't smoke. Spend time walking or exercising together.

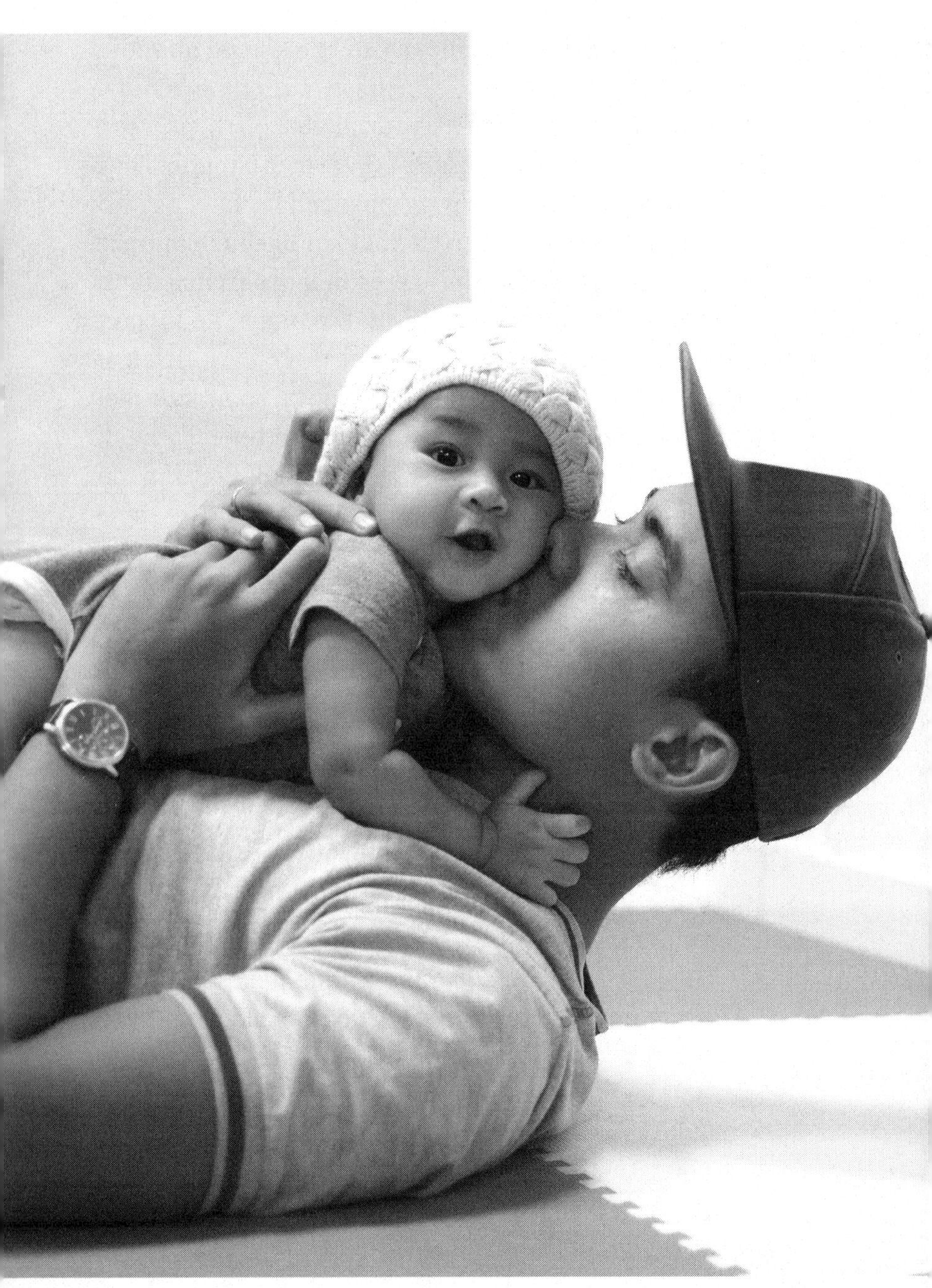

- Try to find ways to cut back on the hours you spend at your workplace, so you have more time at home together.
- Your wife may be intensely demanding. Go with it. She's doing all the heavy lifting. The least you can do is shop for groceries, arrange for paternity leave if you can, so you'll be able to participate in your baby's care during the first days and weeks after birth.
- Changes in desire are common for men and women during this major life change. You probably won't have sex as often as you did before. Perhaps the most common reason men (and women) cut back on their sexual life during pregnancy is a fear that they'll hurt the baby. If you're concerned about that, you can stop worrying right now. The solution here is to talk to each other about how you feel and about your desires and needs.

Of course, you are involved

When you are going to experience the most satisfying desire of your life – fatherhood, you, of course, are involved in the process. However, it is important to express it to your partner also. Expressing your involvement to your partner relieves her tension and apprehensions and gives an essence of security and support.

To be mother also feels happy that all the pain she's taking to be mother is appreciated by you, and you value the sufferings, she is undergoing to fulfil your desire of fatherhood too. It will also make her experience more enjoyable, as she feels that she is giving you the most important desire of life.

Her feeling that you are with her every moment of her journey of motherhood will make you feel very special and strengthen your bond with her. Do not leave this opportunity to help your partner in the most demanding time of her life.

Show that you care

Going to become a father is an equally exciting experience for a man. You know that your wife is taking all the stress and strain of the pregnancy and expected stress and strain of labour and post-natal care to complete your family. You also realise it and are always willing to take care of her and your to-be-born child in the best possible manner. Unfortunately, a man's nature is such that he cannot express his care very effectively. He equally cares for you and your child. A woman's nature is such that she always expects that you show that you care and it is even more important in the times of stress like pregnancy.

It is very easy for you to do it if you try hard enough.

- Ask her daily about how she feels.
- Talk about changes in her body, her emotions, discomforts, difficulties, etc.

You cannot take the physical discomfort and pain away from her, but just by sharing, you relieve them by more than 50%. It really doesn't take a lot of effort.

Prepare or help her prepare the food she loves and encourage her to eat the right food for her and your child.

Try and accompany her to maximum number of her visits to the hospital.

Try and understand the complaints and problems of your wife, the solutions and advice given by the doctor, discuss with your wife about it and help her make a strategy to overcome them.

Your wife doesn't want you to stop your business and stay with her for 24 hours. However, she does expect a little more time with her which you can certainly manage. She may have fear and phobias about the unknown. Gather information about the 'fears' from books, internet or doctors and help her in eliminating them.

Your expression of 'you care' will mean a lot to her. Don't miss this opportunity.

Hey! You are a father now (prepare yourself to be one)

You really are a very happy man when you are becoming a father. It is probably the most satisfying moment in life for a man. Nothing else in the world can give you more joy and satisfaction than becoming a father.

It's the ultimate achievement of your manhood and man's ego. However, this comes with a lot of responsibilities, your responsibility towards the new member of the family and coping up with it, financial burden of your new responsibilities, etc. Your wife is going to be more involved in bringing up the child. Hence, she may dedicate more time and energy to the child. She may not be able to work the same way she did earlier and may not be able to help you in your personal and professional life. You need to understand, cooperate and manage the changed situations to make your experience more fulfilling and enjoyable. It will help the entire family adjust to the changes happily, welcome the newcomer and make everyone's life more pleasurable.

Life is going to change

Arrival of a child in the family changes the life of the entire family, including yours. You would like to bunk your unnecessary appointments and come home early. Your office will close early and you will be restless to reach home just to get a smile or glimpse of your child. A small delicate movement, a tender touch, or non-specific sound of goo-goo or an innocent smile will make you crazy. You will forget worries of your work and fatigue of the day. Do not miss this opportunity as this time will not come back. The small sickness of your child may make the entire family tense and disturbed. Your responsibilities will also increase. You are

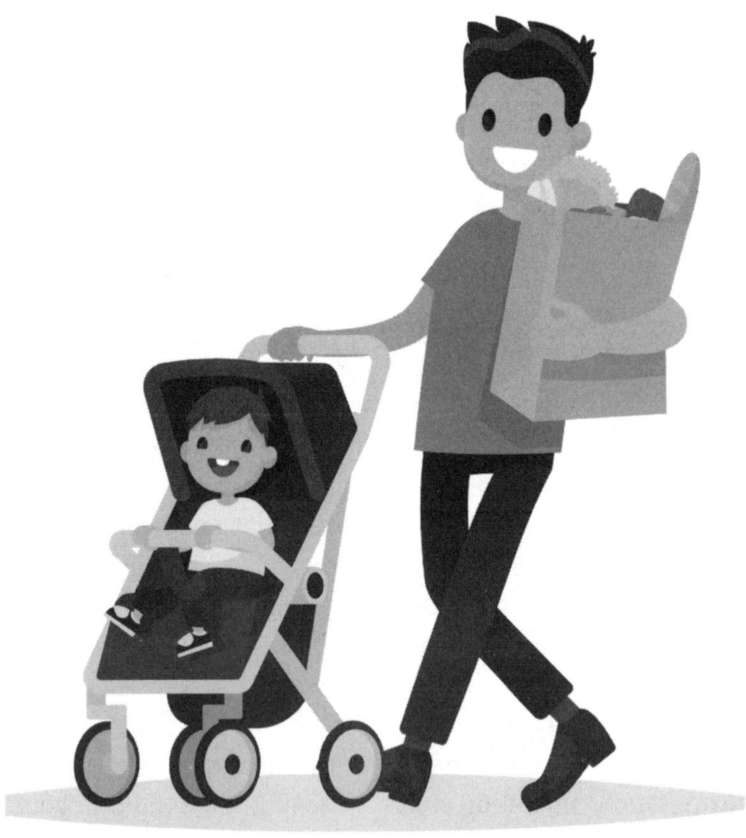

no longer free birds. You cannot plan anything, anytime, but it's a different life, it's a different world.

Welcome to the world of fatherhood. Your world is going to change, your duties, liabilities and responsibilities will be different. Equally different will be your future plans, business plans, investment plans, etc.

Enjoy the difference!

□

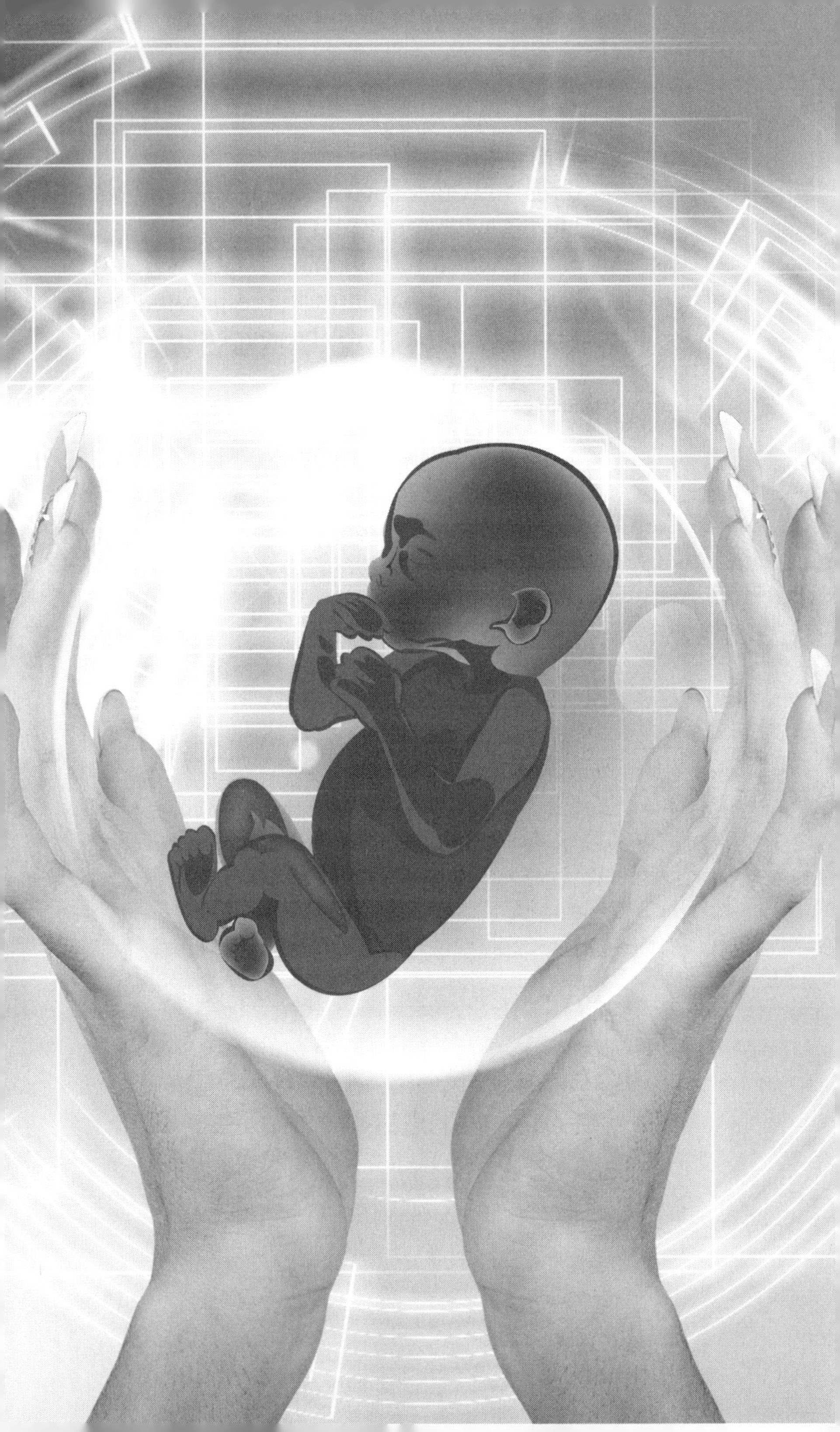

24
Customs and Beliefs

The Indian customs in pregnancy are strictly not followed as before but, however, they are given far more importance than the other customs in our society.

Certain foods are believed to have either a 'cooling' or a 'heating' effect on the functions of various organs of the body, such as mood, personality, and physical well-being. For example, when the mother is breastfeeding, if a baby has a cold or fever, in the former case, she may avoid 'cold' foods and the converse when the baby has a raised temperature. This concept is quite divorced from the actual temperature of food or the intensity of taste of spices. High protein, acid, and salty foods are considered 'hot', whereas 'cold foods' are often sweet. Lentils, eggplant, and grapes are examples of 'hot' foods, and cereals, potatoes, milk, and white sugar are examples of 'cold' foods.

Some common conceptions regarding food are

Myth: Hot foods will cause miscarriage

Fact: This is wrong. It will not cause miscarriage. Hot foods include: Raw papaya, banana, coconut, pineapples, red chilies, eggplant, okra, jackfruit, potatoes, nuts, meat, fish, chicken and eggs.

Myth: Increase in body heat causes morning sickness. The 'Hot Food' causes increase in body heat resulting in nausea, dizziness, swelling of feet and hands.

Fact: This is small rise in temperature during pregnancy which is due to hormonal changes during pregnancy and not due to the hot food

Myth: 'Cold foods' will help with pregnancy

Fact: Pregnancy is considered as a time of increased heat for the woman. Eating cold foods has a cooling effect that is beneficial during pregnancy. Cold foods include: Dairy products, vegetables and fruits that are not hot. 'Cool on stomach' may help reduce pregnancy symptoms.

Myth: Overeating causes problems during labour

Fact: False. It is believed that overeating causes very large foetus, causing complications during labour.

Myth: Ghee, and Butter are good. They provide 'Takat' (Strength)

Fact: Ghee, butter and coconut oil are high in saturated fats and should be avoided in excess amounts for the health of the mother.

They do give calories, but lack in good nutritive substances and, hence, good for physically active women, but others should take it in limited proportion.

Myth: Almonds help in the foetal brain development.

Fact: Almonds are very beneficial for pregnant women as a source of Vitamin E, proteins and folate.

Myth: Consumption of turmeric lightens the skin pigmentation of the unborn.

Fact: Turmeric is an excellent antibiotic, anti-inflammatory, and anti-ulcerative. It increases detoxifying enzymes in the liver, and may lower bad cholesterol levels.

Myth: Papaya can cause miscarriage.

Fact: The white latex in the unripe green papaya can cause miscarriage. However, there is nothing wrong with fully ripened papaya.

Myth: Shape of the mother's stomach tells the gender.

Fact: Tradition says that if her stomach is carrying baby low, it must be a baby boy and if her stomach is carrying baby high, it must be a girl. This popular notion has no scientific basis. The shape and position is determined by the original shape of her abdomen, her uterine muscle tone strength of abdominal muscle and number of Foetus and position of baby.

Myth: Shape of the face and skin tones signifies the gender.

Fact: Have you heard your aunt or grandmother saying that you are going to have a girl because your face looks glowing after you conceive? You should not anticipate anything based on their analysis, because like the other myths, this too does not have a scientific basis. Pregnant women normally have some weight gain during pregnancy that could affect the shape of their faces and skin tones.

Myth: Not to put arms around your head.

Fact: Sometimes women are advised not to put arms around their head, because if they do that, they might risk their baby's strangulation by the umbilical cord. But this belief is baseless, as there is no definite scientific study to confirm this.

Myth: Not to take a bath.

Fact: There is a myth that you should not take bath regularly, when you are pregnant. This too is baseless, since maintaining hygiene is a general requirement during pregnancy.

Myth: Consuming some food items will give a fair complexion.

Fact: Sometimes elders advise you to drink a mixture of saffron and milk or eat oranges during pregnancy to have the child born with a fairer complexion. But this too seems to have little validity, since the skin tone is determined by the genes. Food items have very little to do with the original complexion of your baby.

Some other common beliefs are

There are some wrong beliefs in all those cases; the danger feared is abortion from the influence of evil spirits:

- The pregnant women should never go close to a dead body, even if it's her near relative.

As any sad event can cause sad feelings in any individual, particularly so in females as they are usually more emotional. Death of near one or close relative causes intense sadness and even more negative emotions. Any emotional shocks or stress on a pregnant lady can prove to be detrimental to her and her baby's health. Hence, traditionally a pregnant lady is not allowed to attend funerals and sad events. In ancient times, in the absence of scientific evidence, everything was attributed or talked about as good spirits and evil spirits. But the logic was to keep a mother-to-be happy and safe. In modern times, the decision in such things can be taken on a case-to-case basis depending upon the personality of the pregnant lady and all other circumstances.

- She should never cross a stream, especially in the dark or in the evenings, or else the water spirit can cast an evil influence on her.

This again is to safeguard the mother in those times where the facility to cross a river and light were not as they arc today.

- The pregnant woman should not visit a woman who has delivered a child recently.

Labour pain and childbirth are very painful processes. There is always a small chance of complications. Every lady has a different tolerance level, every individual is different and every labour is different. Hence, scary talks about experience of childbirth may scare a pregnant lady about childbirth process. Hygiene was also very difficult during menses and postnatal period in ancient times. Hence, it was considered unhygienic to go to a lady during her menses or postnatal period. In the postnatal period, the mother is recovering from stress and pain of labour and related procedures, if any, and bonding with the child, breastfeeding and taking care of all its requirements. Hence, she needs enough time, rest and privacy for the same. Hence, in modern times, though the above-mentioned situations have drastically changed, care must be taken not to allow negative experiences of a delivered lady (postnatal period) to affect the pregnant lady. Hence, decision has to be taken on case-to-case basis.

- If a snake appears in front of the woman and tries to escape, it confirms her pregnancy.

There is no such scientific basis.

- The people believed that the shadow of a pregnant woman falling on a snake will cause it to crawl slowly in any other direction.

There is no such scientific basis.

- During pregnancy, both the parents are vulnerable to the effects of an eclipse. Thus, it is safest for the wife to stay indoors and not even catch a glimpse of the eclipse. But the father is not under any such strict prohibitions.

The actual effect of eclipse is a matter of research for a scientist. Though care must be taken by everybody while watching an eclipse, specific ill effects on a pregnant lady are not proven.

- A premature birth in the eighth month of pregnancy is sometimes superstitiously attributed to a cat having entered the mother's room in a 'former' confinement. It is believed by some that a child born in this month could die on the eighth day, in the eighth month, the eighth year, or the eighteenth year! Some Hindus, therefore, consider the number "eight" unlucky. A child born in the seventh month of pregnancy has better chances of survival than a child born in eight month of pregnancy.

This is a false belief. More maturity is always beneficial for survival of a child. A child born after seventh or eighth month can survive; if required, the decision of delivering a child should be taken based on benefits and risks of waiting.

□

25
Postnatal Care

Postnatal period is the period beginning immediately after the birth of a baby and extending for about 6 weeks. It is the time after birth in which the mother's body, including hormone level and uterus size, returns to normal non-pregnant state.

Changes in you after the birth of your baby

- Your tummy will feel soft and round; you won't look pregnant but your tummy won't resemble the pre-pregnancy state either. Within minutes of delivery, the uterus (womb) changes from a sac with a capacity to hold four-and-a-half litres of liquid to a grapefruit-sized pouch of muscle. The uterus will downsize in weight from 1000 g to 50 g within six weeks.
- You will feel some 'after pains' in your uterus when breastfeeding because it is shrinking in size.
- The vaginal muscles will slowly regain its former tone and the pelvic floor will return to its previous position. Tears to the neck of the womb, vagina and perineum should also heal quickly.

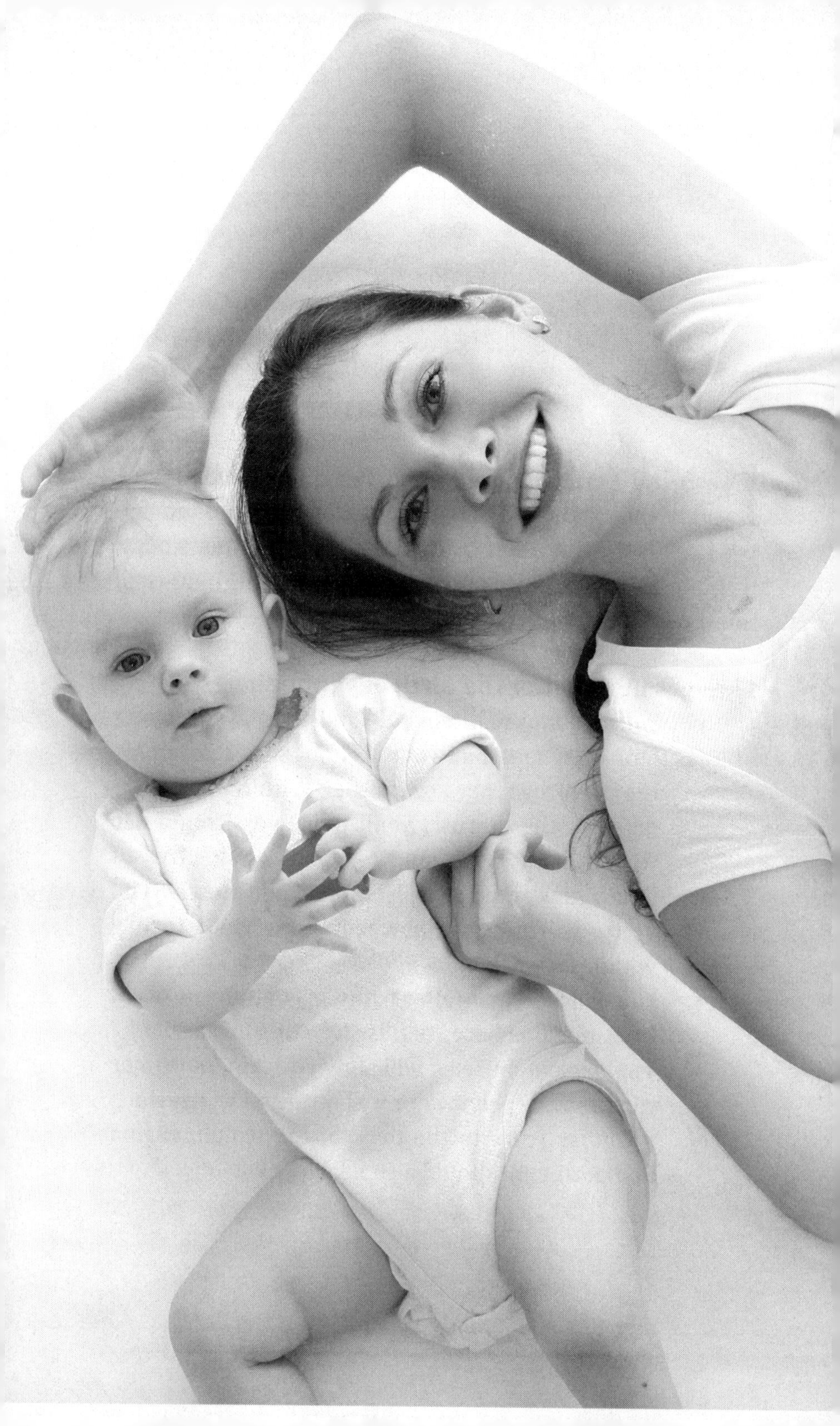

- Your breasts grow bigger from day 2 or 3 as 'milk comes in'. Slight feeling of discomfort is normal but this is temporary.
- After childbirth, progesterone levels fall rapidly causing discomforts, such as heartburn, constipation and varicose veins, although haemorrhoids (piles) take longer to resolve.
- In the first few weeks, there will be a lot of vaginal discharge. The uterus is shedding the rest of its lining. This discharge, or lochia, is red in the start. It changes to pinkish brown and then cream. Use sanitary towels and avoid tampons, as there's a risk of infection. Heart, lungs and circulation, relieved of the burden of pregnancy, assume normalcy gradually.
- Joints of the pelvis and spine, softened by the hormones during pregnancy take time to get back to normal. Back discomfort may continue for months to come, so be cautious with lifting and carrying. Best to avoid heavy stuff. The abdominal muscles, stretched to twice their normal length during pregnancy, regain their tone within a couple of months. Getting back to your pre-pregnancy weight and appearance takes time.
- Weight loss is most rapid and obvious in the first few days after delivery as the extra two to eight litres of water carried during late pregnancy are passed out as urine. Thereafter, weight loss slows down. Exercising and eating right will help in later months.
- Some leg and ankle swelling may begin during the first two days after delivery and can persist for

several weeks. This is not unusual. When resting, reading or watching TV, elevate your legs using pillows or cushions above the level of your hips. If your legs remain painful and swollen, call your caregiver.

- Occasionally you will feel tired and weepy – it is normal to go through this. Don't confuse this with postnatal depression.

Your first check-up post delivery

This is your last visit to your obstetrician (the 6th week check-up) where you will receive a thorough check-up. Basically your doctor will want to make sure your body is healing well after the delivery of your baby.

- Your weight will be taken and your blood pressure will be measured.
- A pelvic exam to assess if your uterus is getting back to its pre-pregnancy size, your cervix is closed and the episiotomy has healed well.
- Checks stitches, if any.
- A check of your emotional and overall well being.
- Advice on minor problems such as constipation and birth control.

Now is the time to make life easier

- Accept any offers of help. Hire a temporary help if you must, since it is easily available anywhere. You may need all the help you can get in the initial phase for the basics around the house, i.e., cooking, cleaning up, shopping etc.
- Visitors will come pouring in to visit you and your baby. Since this is especially customary in any

culture, it becomes all the more necessary to make it safe for you and the baby.

- Don't forget your pelvic floor exercises – you can start these as soon as you like, even from the first day after the birth. If you have concerns on exercising, address them with your doctor.
- You may lose up to twelve pounds when the baby is born and maybe another one or two the following week. If you continue to follow the healthy eating habits suggested during pregnancy, the weight should come off naturally. Crash diet is not the solution, especially if you are breastfeeding. Talk to your caregiver about healthy weight loss. Breastfeeding moms should aim for four servings of milk and milk products each day. To make sure you get all the nutrients, you need when you first get home, let someone else cook for you.
- Ignore the need to get back to normalcy just after coming home from the hospital. If you feel like staying in your night clothes all day, do it. Everything takes time; don't pressurise yourself. The key issue is rest. The more you rest and take care of yourself in the first few weeks, the quicker you will return to your normal self.

When your doctor has assured you on your full recovery, join a postnatal exercise class. This is a really good way of making friends and keeping fit. Alternatively, you can engage in more strenuous abdominal exercises like sit-ups and curl-ups at home. These exercises may help you flatten your stomach and lose weight. Bear in mind, it takes up to three months for your body to recover from the birth.

Postnatal care includes some pelvic floor exercises

- Pull up around the vagina as if to stop urinating. Hold for a count of four and release. You should feel the difference when you let go.
- Repeat the exercise in batches of six or eight as often as you can during the day.
- As well as holding for a count of four, try doing some where you squeeze, release, squeeze, release quite quickly.
- Breathe normally throughout the exercise. As soon as possible after delivery, start doing pelvic floor exercises. If you have stitches, you will be sore, but the exercise will improve your circulation and help your perineum heal. If you have had a caesarean, you will still need to do your pelvic floor exercises.

Pelvic rock

- Lie on your back with knees bent and feet flat on the floor. As you breathe out, rock your pelvis so that the small of your back flattens onto the floor. Then rock your pelvis again so that your back is lifted away from the floor.

Leg slide

- Lie on your back, knees bent and feet flat on the floor. Put your hand in the small of your back, flat against the floor. As you breathe out, let your legs slide forward slowly, bringing your knees closer to the ground. Then gently slide your legs up again.

Some points to observe

- Start with gentle exercises in the first few weeks after the birth. Follow the clues your body gives you.
- Do not lie flat on your back and lift both legs in the air.

- Do not lie flat on your back and do sit-ups with your feet held down.
- If in doubt, wait till you go for your check up and consult your doctor on the dos and don'ts of exercise.

Breastfeeding your baby

Hormonal changes after delivery prompt your breasts to start producing milk. When your baby nurses during the first few days after birth, he/she is getting colostrum, a thick yellowish substance that your breasts produce during pregnancy. His/her suckling triggers the release of the hormones prolactin, which stimulates milk production, and oxytocin, which causes the milk sacs and ducts to contract, propelling the milk to your nipples. (This is the so-called 'let-down' reflex.)

If in the first breastfeeding sessions, you feel some abdominal cramping, it's because oxytocin also triggers uterine contractions. When your milk comes in, usually two to three days after you give birth, your breasts may get swollen, tender, hard, throbbing, and uncomfortably full. This is called engorgement and it should get better in a day or two.

Nursing your baby often is the best thing you can do for relief.

Diet

One of the wonders of breast milk is that it can meet your baby's nutritional needs even when you're not eating perfectly. However, if your diet is too low in calories or relies on one food group at the exclusion of others, this could affect the quality and quantity of your milk.

When you don't get the nutrients you need from your diet, your body draws on its reserves, which can eventually become depleted. Also, you need strength and stamina to meet the physical demands of caring for a new baby.

Eating a mix of carbohydrates, protein and fat at meals keep you feeling full longer and supplies the nutrients your body needs. Complex carbohydrates like whole grains and cereals and fresh fruits and vegetables not only provide more nutrition than processed starches and sugars, they provide lasting energy.

Limit saturated fats and avoid trans-fats, both of which are unhealthy. Saturated fats show up in high-fat meats, whole milk, tropical oils (such as palm kernel and coconut) and butter.

Drink plenty of fluid. A good guideline to follow is drink to satisfy thirst – that is, drink whenever you feel the need. If your urine is clear or light yellow, it's a good sign that you're well hydrated. Nursing moms should limit their consumption of caffeine.

Some moms feel that certain foods – like cabbage, dairy products, chocolate, citrus, garlic, or chili pepper – make their breastfed baby gassy or irritable. If your baby seems consistently uncomfortable after you eat a particular food, then by all means, avoid it to see if your baby is happier.

Body changes

You probably won't return to your pre-pregnancy weight for some time, but you will lose a significant amount of weight immediately after delivery. Subtracting weight of the baby, placenta, and of the blood and amniotic fluid leaves most new moms about 6-7 kg lighter.

The weight keeps coming off too. All the extra water your cells retained during pregnancy, along with fluid from the extra blood you had in your pregnant body, will be looking for a way out.

Lose your pregnancy weight gradually. Plan to take up to a year to get back to your pre-pregnancy weight.

If you give birth vaginally, your vagina will probably remain a little larger than it was before. Right after delivery, the vagina will be stretched open and may be swollen and bruised. Over the next few days, any swelling you might have starts to go down, and your vagina begins to regain muscle tone. In the next few weeks, it will gradually get smaller. Doing Kegel exercises regularly helps restore muscle tone.

If you had a small tear in your perineum that did not require stitches, it should heal quickly and cause little discomfort. If you had an episiotomy or a significant tear, your perineum needs time to heal.

Wait to start having sex again until you get the okay from your doctor at your postpartum check-up at 6 weeks after delivery. If you continue to have tenderness in that area, delay intercourse until you feel ready.

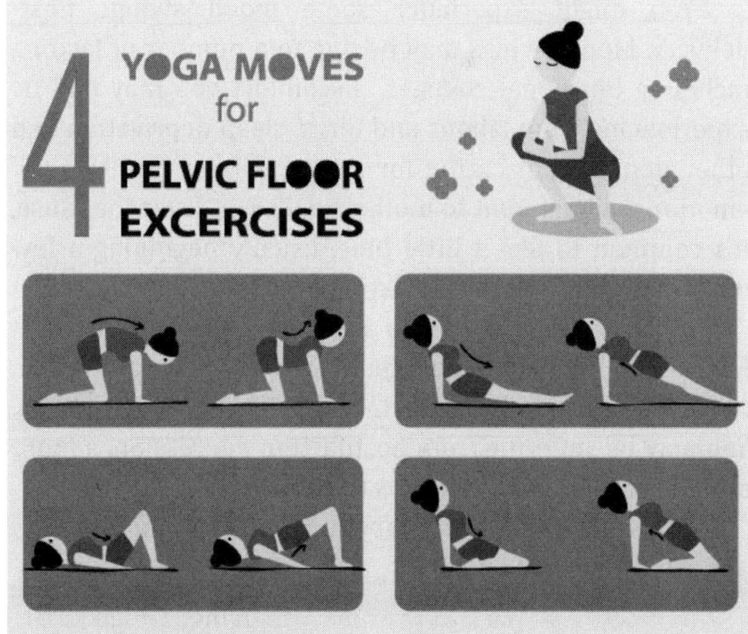

In the meantime, figure out what you want to do for contraception. When you do feel ready (both physically and emotionally) to have sex again, be sure to go slow.

It's normal to have vaginal discharge, called lochia, for a month or two after you give birth. Lochia consists of blood, bacteria and sloughed-off tissue from the lining of the uterus.

For the first few days after birth, the lochia contains a fair amount of blood, so it will be bright red and look like a heavy menstrual period. You'll likely have a bit less discharge each day, and by two to four days, after you've given birth, the lochia will be more watery and pinkish in colour.

After about ten days you've given birth, you'll have only a small amount of white or yellow-white discharge, which will taper off over the next two to four weeks.

You might experience some mood swings post-delivery. Mood swings may be due to a number of factors, including hormonal changes, discomfort you may still be experiencing from labour and birth, sleep deprivation and other demands of caring for a new baby, as well as the emotional adjustment to motherhood. Whatever the cause, it's common to feel a little blue, usually beginning a few days after giving birth and lasting for a few weeks.

If the feeling doesn't go away on its own in the first few weeks or you find that you're feeling worse rather than better, be sure to call your doctor and tell her your symptoms. You may be suffering from postpartum depression, a more serious problem that requires treatment.

You should take your baby for routine immunisations as advised by your doctor.

In case of any of these danger signs mentioned below you should contact your doctor immediately:

Danger signs for the mother

- Excessive bleeding
- Foul-smelling vaginal discharge
- Fever with or without chills
- Severe abdominal pain
- Excessive tiredness or breathlessness
- Swollen hands, face and legs with severe headaches or blurred vision
- Painful, engorged breasts or sore, cracked, bleeding nipples

Danger signs for the baby

- Convulsions
- Movement only when stimulated or no movement, even when stimulated, not feeding well
- Fast breathing (more than 60 breaths per minute), grunting or severe chest in-drawing
- Fever (above 38°C)
- Low body temperature (below 35.5°C),
- Very small baby (less than 1500 grams or born more than two months early)

□

26

Cord Blood/Stem Cell Preservation

What are stem cells?

Stem Cells are master cells whose definite function in the body is determined only after they receive signals directing them to become specific cell types. Because of their ability to specialise as any cells of a human body, stem cells are used as the BASIC BUILDING MATERIAL in the body's constant renewal process.

What types of stem cells are there in the umbilical cord?

The blood that remains in the umbilical cord, after it is separated at the time of delivery, is a rich source of haematopoietic (blood forming) stem cells (HSCs). The umbilical cord tissue, often referred to as Wharton's Jelly, acts as a source of mesenchymal (Tissue and Organ forming) stem cells (MSCs).

What are the uses of these stem cells?

These HSCs (Haematopoietic Stem Cells) are being successfully used to cure diseases like leukemia, thalassaemia, sickle cell anaemia, fanconi's anaemia and many more life-threatening blood disorders. Against laks of stem cell samples stored, approximately 30,000 cord blood transplants have been done with variable success.

These MSCs (Mesenchymal Stem Cells) have enormous potential to facilitate repair and regenerate normal tissue function. Scientists predict new therapies using MSCs being available and universally adopted. This may include treatment for cerebral palsy, autism, type 1 diabetes, etc.

What makes it special and different than an adult stem cell?

Umbilical cord stem cells are biologically younger and more flexible compared to adult stem cells from bone marrow and other sources. It has unique qualities and advantages like:

- Less risk of complications when used for transplant latins.
- Ability to use one's own stem cells for conditions that currently lack medical treatment – this option is known as 'autologous transplantation'.
- Immediate availability and minimise disease progression by early treatment.
- Stem cell is useful not only for the baby, but it may also be useful to parents, siblings, family members or any matching recipient.

Limitations of stem cell preservation

- Treatment success is limited except for haematological disorder.
- May not be sufficient for complete therapy.
- Very less percentage of stored samples is actually used.
- Does not guarantee a cure.

Couples should understand cost vs. benefits of stem cell preservation and then make their choice. Decision must be made before delivery as once we discard cord and placenta, we cannot recover the stem cells.

□

27
Newborn Screening

Newborn Screening

What is Newborn Screening?

Newborn screening is the test of child immediately after birth to diagnose certain problematic or life threatening disorder that cannot be seen on examination at birth.

What is the purpose of Newborn Screening?

The purpose of the test is to try to find babies that have these rare and fatal problems in newborn babies before they lead to an irreversible damage to mental and/or physical development and above all, ensure that the treatment is initiated in time so that they may live a better and healthy life.

Newborn screening is recommended by medical councils across the world and is mandatory for all babies born in countries such as UK, USA, Germany, Japan, Australia & several others countries.

How is it be done?

It's a very simple. Just a few drops of blood are collected on filter paper and dried. Baby's heel is pricked with very fine needle. It's not a painful procedure.

What is the chance of detecting a condition?

The chance of detecting a particular condition is very less, however the chances of detection also depends on the number of diseases are being tested.

Normally, a baby can be screened for at least 57 diseases with this technique.

But all babies need not be screened for all diseases. All babies should be screened for at least 6 common diseases which are not evident initially and which have treatment if diagnosed in time. These diseases are Congenital Hypothyroidism, G6 PD deficiency, Congenital Adrenal Hyperplasia, Galactosemia, Phenylketonurea, and Biotinidase deficiency.

What if the test is abnormal?

An abnormal result may indicate the need for a second test to diagnose a condition. Further, if the condition is diagnosed, an early medical intervention will play a key role in helping the baby lead a normal life.

What is the sensitivity of this test?

Newborn screening tests provide an early opportunity to detect certain conditions – before symptoms appear.

However, we know that even the best screening cannot always detect a condition. Moreover, a screening test is limited to the conditions included in its scope. There are many more conditions which may have similar manifestations.

If your baby does not seem well, talk to your baby's doctor as soon as possible.

□

28
Immunization Schedule

Age completed weeks/ months/ years	Vaccines	Comments
Birth	BCG, OPV 0 Hep-B 1	Administer these vaccines to all newborns before hospital discharge
6 weeks	DTwP 1, IPV 1 Hep-B 2, Hib 1 Rotavirus 1, PCV 1	**DTP:** • DTaP vaccine/combinations should preferably be avoided for the primary series • DTaP vaccine/ combinations should be preferred in certain specific circumstances/conditions only • No need of repeating/giving additional doses of whole-cell pertussis (wP) vaccine to a child who has earlier completed their primary schedule with acellular pertussis (aP) vaccine-containing products

		Polio: • All doses of IPV may be replaced with OPV if administration of the former is unfeasible • Additional doses of OPV on all supplementary immunisation activities (SIAs) • Two doses of IPV instead of 3 for primary series if started at 8 weeks, and 8 weeks interval between the doses • No child should leave the facility without polio immunisation (IPV or OPV), if indicated by the schedule • See footnotes under figure tiled IAP recommended immunisation schedule (with range) for recommendations on intradermal IPV **Rotavirus:** 2 doses of RV1 and 3 doses of RV5 & RV 116E • RV1 should be employed in 10 & 14 week schedule, 10 & 14 week schedule of RV1 is found to be more immunogenic than 6 & 10 week schedule
10 weeks	DTwP 2, IPV 2 Hib 2, Rotavirus 2 PCV 2	**Rotavirus** If RV1 is chosen, the first dose should be given at 10 weeks

14 weeks	DTwP 3, IPV 3 Hib 3, Rotavirus 3 PCV 3	**Rotavirus** • Only 2 doses of RV1 are recommended. • If RV1 is chosen, the 2nd dose should be given at 14 week
6 months	OPV 1 Hep-B 3	**Hepatitis-B** The final (3rd or 4th) dose in the HepB vaccine series should be administered no earlier than age 24 weeks and at least 16 weeks after the first dose.
9 months	OPV 2 MMR-1	**Hepatitis-B** • Measles-containing vaccine ideally should not be administered before completing 270 days or 9 months • The 2nd dose must follow in 2nd year of life • No need to give stand-alone measles vaccine
9-12 months	Typhoid Conjugate Vaccine	• Currently, two typhoid conjugate vaccines, Typbar-TCV® and PedaTyph® available in Indian market; either can be used • An interval of at least 4 weeks with the MMR vaccine should be maintained while administering this vaccine
12 months	Hep-A 1	**Hepatitis-A:** • Single dose for live attenuated H2-strain Hep-A vaccine • Two doses for all inactivated Hep-A vaccines are recommended

15 months	MMR 2 Varicella 1 PCV booster	**MMR:** • The 2nd dose must follow in 2nd year of life • However, it can be given at anytime 4-8 weeks after the 1st dose Varicella: The risk of breakthrough varicella is lower if given 15 months onwards
16-18 months	DTwP B1/ DTaP B1 IPV B1 Hib B1	The first booster (4th dose) may be administered as early as age 12 months, provided at least 6 months have elapsed since the third dose **DTP:** • First & second boosters should preferably be of DTwP • Considering a higher reactogenicity of DTwP, DTaP can be considered for the boosters
18 months	Hep-A 2	**Hepatii A:** 2nd dose for inactivated vaccines only
2 year	Booster of Typhoid Conjugate Vaccine	• A booster dose of Typhoid conjugate vaccine (TCV), if primary dose is given at 9-12 months • A dose of Typhoid Vi-polysaccharide (Vi-PS) vaccine can be given if conjugate vaccine is not available or feasible; • Revaccination every 3 years with Vi-polysaccharide vaccine

<table>
<tr><td></td><td></td><td>• Typhoid conjugate vaccine should be preferred over Vi-PS vaccine</td></tr>
<tr><td>4 to 6 year</td><td>DTwP B2/
DTaP
B2
OPV 3
Varicella 2
MMR 3</td><td>Varicella:
the 2nd dose can be given at anytie 3 months after the 1st dose.
MMR:
the 3rd dose is recommended at 4-6 years of age.</td></tr>
<tr><td>10 to 12 year</td><td>Tdap/Td
HPV</td><td>Tdap:
is preferred to Td followed by Td every 10 years</td></tr>
<tr><td colspan="3">HPV:
• Only 2 doses of either of the two HPV vaccines for adolescent/preadolescent girls aged 9-14 years
• For girls 15 years and older, and immunocompromised individuals 3 doses are recommended
• For two-dose schedule, the minimum interval between doses should be 6 months</td></tr>
<tr><td colspan="3">• For 3 dose schedule, the doses can be administered at 0, 1-2 (depending on brand) and 6 months</td></tr>
<tr><td colspan="3">Recommended vaccines for High-risk children (Vaccines under special circumstances):
• Influenza Vaccine, Meningococcal Vaccine
• Japanese Encephalitis Vaccine, Cholera Vaccine
• Rabies Vaccine, Yellow Fever Vaccine
• Pneumococcal Polysaccharide vaccine (PPSV 23)</td></tr>
</table>

□

Brief introduction to the Contributors

Dr. Himanshu Bavishi

M.D. (Ob &Gyn)

He is a senior Obstetrician and Gynecologist practicing since the last 30 years. As an infertility & IVF specialist he has a vast experience of managing pregnancies and child birth, particularly for precious and high risk pregnancies. He is a co-founder of World recognised and India's leading Fertility Institute – Bavishi Fertility Institute.

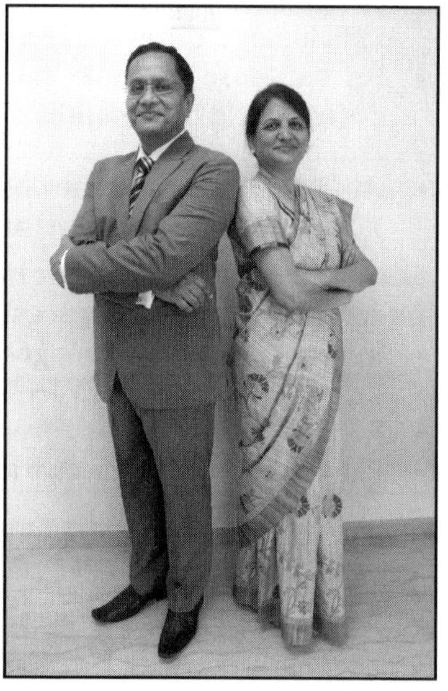

Dr. Falguni Bavishi

M.D. (Ob & Gyn)

She is a senior Obstetrician and Gynecologist practicing since 29 years. She is an infertility and IVF specialist with special skills and knowledge of intricate and high technology IVF Lab procedures. She is the co-founder of – Bavishi Fertility Institute.

Brief introduction to the Contributors

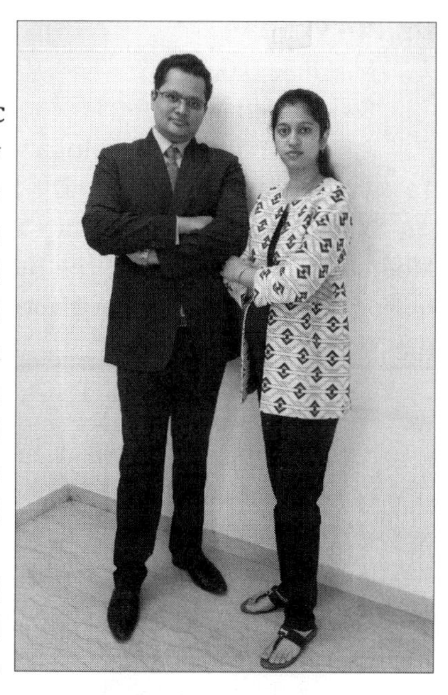

Dr. Parth Bavishi

M.D. (Ob & Gyn)

A young and dynamic institute 'Bavishi Fertility Institute'. He obtained his master's degree from reputed Pramukh Swami Medical College and completed his fellowship & special infertility training in Foetal Medicine and Obstetric Ultrasound from NHL Municipal Medical College.

He has obtained special training at Diamond Institute for infertility and Menopause, USA and Hiroshima Assisted Reproductive Technique Institute, Japan. He is working with Bavishi Fertility Institute since 2012.

Dr. Janki Bavishi

M.S. (Ob & Gyn)

An enthusiastic and sincere specialist she joined the family Institute 'Bavishi Fertility Institute'. She obtained her master's degree from one of the oldest medical college and biggest hospital of Asia, B. J. Medical College. After master degree in Ob & Gy she has contributed enormously to Bavishi Fertility Institute since 2013. She did her specialty infertility training at Diamond Institute for Infertility and Menopause, USA and Hiroshima Assisted Reproductive Technique Institute, Japan.

Brief introduction to the contributors

Dr. Purvi Shah

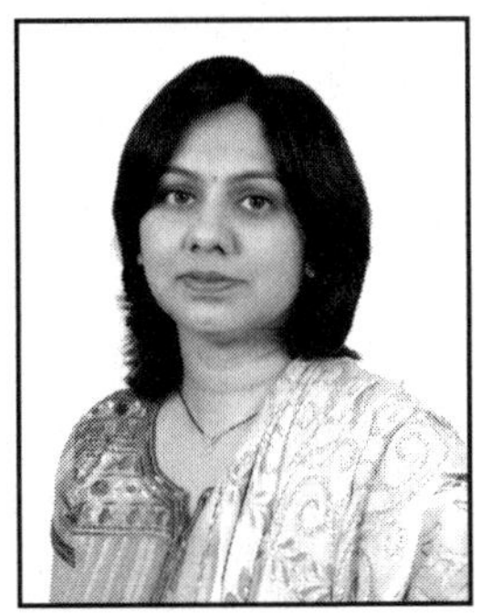

M.B.B.S., D.G.O.

Fellowship in Obstetric ultrasound

A dynamic gynaecologist with 14 years experience and having special training and fellowship in Fetal Medicine. She is a part of the dynamic team of Bavishi Fertility Institute since the last nine years.

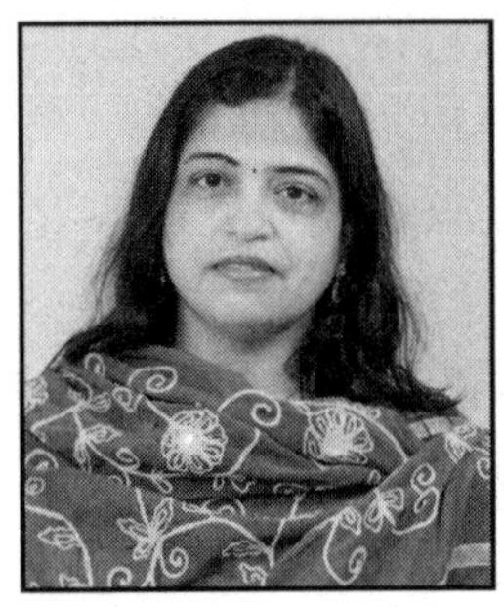

Dr. Binal Shah
MBBS, DGO

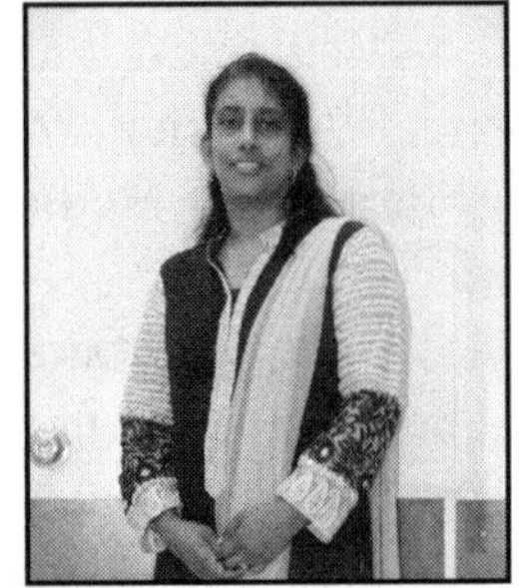

Dr. Lekshmy Rana
MD, DGO, MRCOG

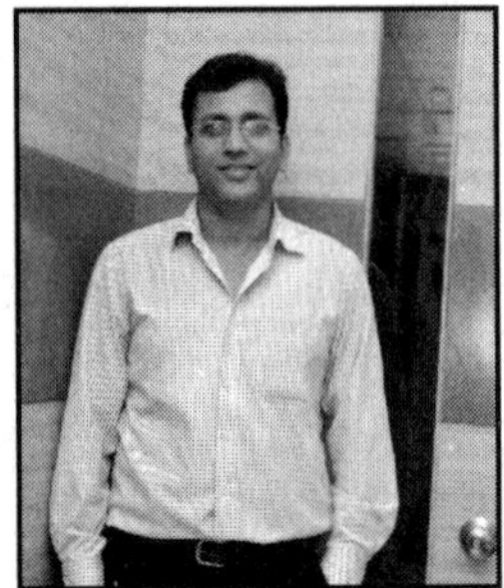

Dr. Sushil Shinde
MBBS, MS

About Bavishi Fertility Institute

The Institute

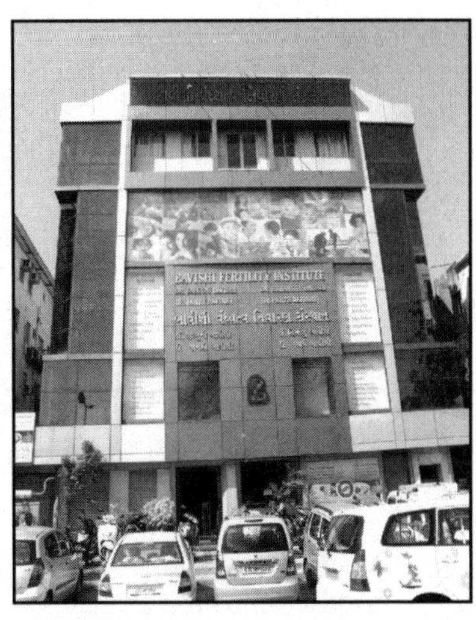

Bavishi fertility institute was established in 1986, as a maternity hospital. Continuous expansion and modernization has made it one the most prestigious fertility institute of India and the World. Today, BFI is India's biggest fertility institute and does one of the highest numbers of infertility treatment procedures and IVF treatment cycles.

A strong team of more than 100 experienced, qualified and dedicated people, including 18 consultants, embryologists, IVF programme coordinators, counsellors, nurses and supporting staff, help BFI maintain very high standard of quality and care. Together we achieve a very high success rate and patient satisfaction.

Our ethics and transparency coupled with commitment and innovation match with our motto -

'Technology • Trust': Now the BFI team has Experience and Enthusiasm Coupled with Wisdom and Vision.

Facilities: Spread over 7 stories and 21,000 Sq. Ft. of space, BFI, has separate floors for different departments.

Infertility: BFI offers all treatment options including, Endoscopy (Laparoscopy – Hysteroscopy), IUI, IVF, ICSI, Assisted hatching, Blastocyst culture, PGS, PGD, Egg/Embryo/ Sperm donation, Egg/ Embryo/Sperm freezing and Surrogate mother.

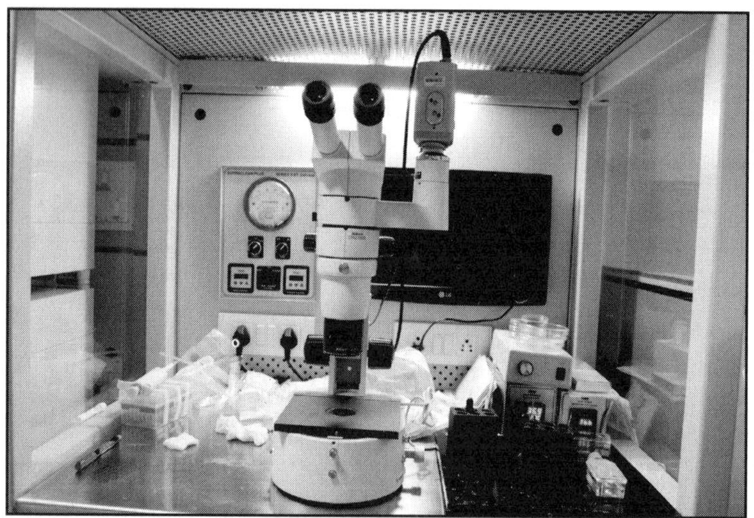

Foetal Medicine and High Risk Pregnancy: Dedicated foetal medicine unit has years of experience in managing high risk and complicated pregnancies, i.e. twins, triplets or higher order multiple gestations, hypertension, gestational diabetes, growth restricted foetuses, preterm labour pain, etc. We offer following services for at risk foetus:

- Prenatal diagnosis of genetic anomalies.
- Prenatal treatment of foetal anomalies.
- Foetal therapy including intrauterine foetal therapies
- Foetal surveillance

Bavishi Fertility Institute, Mumbai

Established in October 2010, BFI MUMBAI is located at one of the most well connected central and posh areas of Mumbai Ghatkopar East. BFI Mumbai, offers all fertility services of the same standards under direct supervision of BFI Ahmedabad. To increase the convenience of people of Mumbai, BFI Mumbai has 5 sub centres at Borivali, Villeparle, Andheri, Dadar, Vashi and Thane. Couples can get all services at these sub centres. Women alone can easily continue their treatment making it much more convenient and sustainable. A team of 4 fertility expert gynecologists - Dr. Lekshmy Rana, Dr. Sushil Shinde, Dr. Riddhi Doshi take care of the centres along with a team of embryologist, counsellors, nurses and support staff. Dr. Falguni Bavishi and Dr. Himanshu Bavishi regularly visit BFI Mumbai to take care of ovum pick up, embryo transfer, consultation & monitoring of all operations. BFI has shifted to a bigger and better facility in 201 7.

Bavishi Bhagat Fertility Institute, Delhi

Bavishi Bhagat Fertility Institute, Delhi, is state of ART-IVF center promoted by Bavishi Fertility Institute Ahmedabad and Delhi's experienced and expert gynecologist Dr. Upasana Bhagat. The institute is located at an ultra modern multi specialty 100 bed hospital, Bhagat Chandra Hospital. Established in September 2009, Bavishi Bhagat Fertility Institute is located in a prime area of Delhi, Dwarka. It is in proximity to domestic and International airport. BBFI Delhi offers all fertility services of the same standards as BFI Ahmedabad. Senior consultant Dr. Upasana Bhagat along with a dedicated team is taking care of the centre. Dr. Himanshu Bavishi regularly visits BBFI Delhi for ovum pick up, embryo transfer, and smooth functioning of the institute. BBFI offers all fertility treatments under one roof. Located in the capital of India, BBFI Delhi is also becoming a preferred destination for IVF treatment from people across the globe.

Bavishi Pratiksha Fertility Institute, Kolkata

Bavishi Pratiksha Fertility Institute, is state-of-art IVF center promoted by Bavishi Fertility Institute, Pratiksha Group of Hospitals and Srishti Hospitals. The ultra-modern Institute is spread across more than 8000 sq feet and two floors and is located in a prime area of Kolkata. BPFI, Kolkata offers all fertility services of world class standards and care.

A qualified team of consultants, embryologists and other staff take care of patient's needs. The centre is designed and made as per the highest standards of medical care and focused on specific needs of infertility management services. BPFI offers various, most reasonable 'Value for money' price packages to suit the budget of every couple. BPFI Kolkata is the preferred destination for fertility treatment for couples of West Bengal and other neighbouring states and countries.

Bavishi Fertility Institute, Surat

Bavishi Fertility Institute Surat, was established in 2009. It is located in a prime area of Surat, near the railway station in Param Doctor House. A qualified team of Dr. Aashita Jain, Dr. Dipen Prajapati, Dr. Disha Sakariya (MO) take care of the patients of Surat and it's vicinity, under the dedicated supervision of Dr. Himanshu Bavishi, Dr. Falguni Bavishi and their team of Bavishi Fertility Institute, Ahmedabad.

BFI Surat, offers all fertility services with the latest technology under one roof. The centre is designed and made as per the highest standards of medical care and focused on specific needs of infertility management services.

Publications

For Medical Fraternity

IUI book written by Dr. Falguni and Dr. Himanshu Bavishi for consultant gynaecologist and pathologist for Assisted Reproductive Technique called IUI. 3rd edition was published in 2007

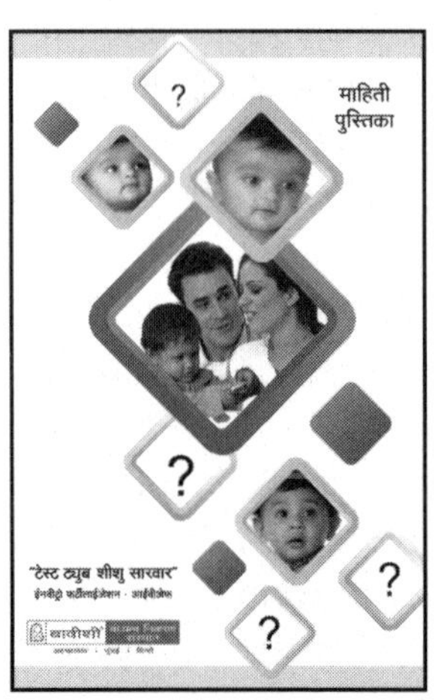

For People

Dev Na Didhela Mangine Lidhela: A unique and first of its kind book of life stories of parents of

222 IVF babies written by parents themselves!

Vighna Dod: The book discusses various dilemma, stress, psychological aspects and more related to infertility treatment. Written by Shri Amrutbhai Patel who has passed through this painful journey of infertility treatment.

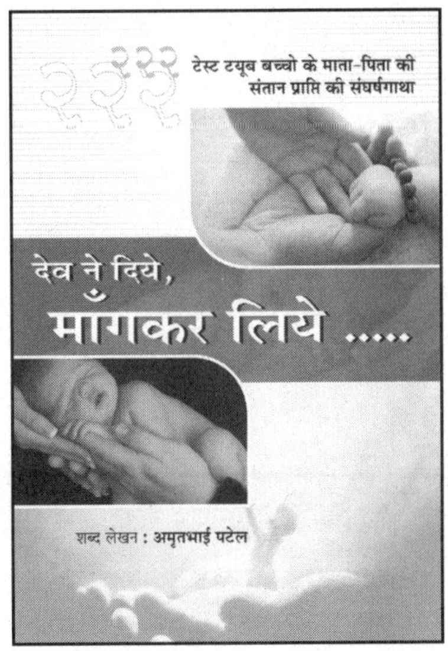

Patient Information Series: Small booklet written in simple and easy language on various infertility problems and treatment options, available in Gujarati, Hindi and English (Marathi coming soon).

Educational Activities

For Medical Fraternity

- BFI has organized many training sessions on various subjects for gynaecologists and other doctors.
- BFI has organized many national and international level conferences, CMEs, workshops and round table meets.

For People

- Interactive patient counselling seminars: 2005, 2012
- Jan Jagruti Abhiyan : in 12 cities, October 2013-February 2014

Social Services

Divya Santan Sansthan and patient support group, 'Divya Santan Parivar'. 'Parivar Milan'

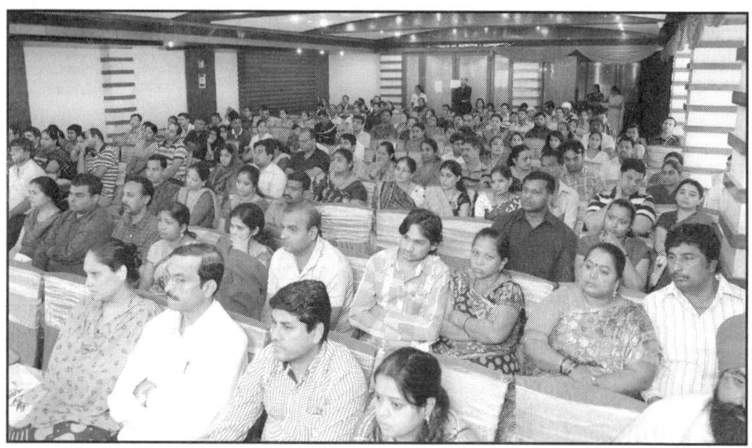

Education and research

- Jan Jagruti Abhiyan 'Public Awareness Programs'
- Bavishi Fertility Institute supports 'Divya Santan Sansthan' for all its activities for providing 'Information Guidance, Inspiration and Solace' through its massive 'Parivar Milan' Abhiyaan and many more activities.

Divya Santan Parivar

- A unique concept for the fist time in India, of support group by successful couples for couples trying to conceive.
- Thousands of people have benefited from this mission in more than 694 events across India, till June 201 6.

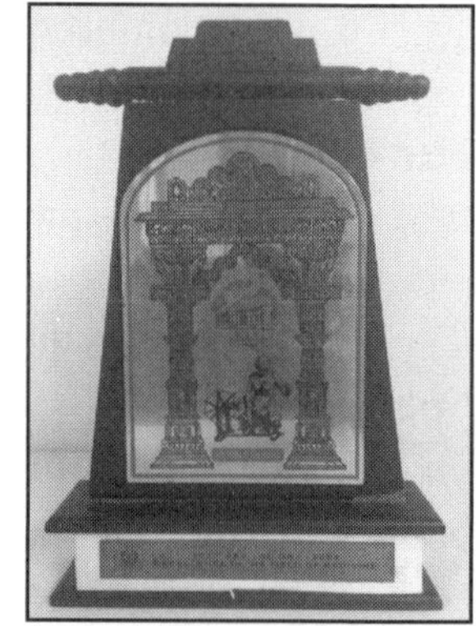

Awards & Milestones

Award Form IMA: Dr. Himanshu Bavishi is the fist IVF specialist to get "Excellence in the Field of Medicine" award from Indian Medical Association, Gujarat State Branch for his pioneering work in the field of infertility

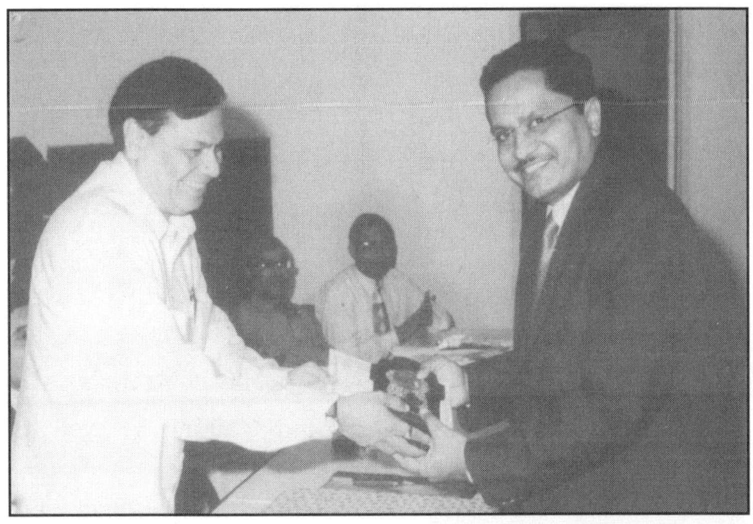

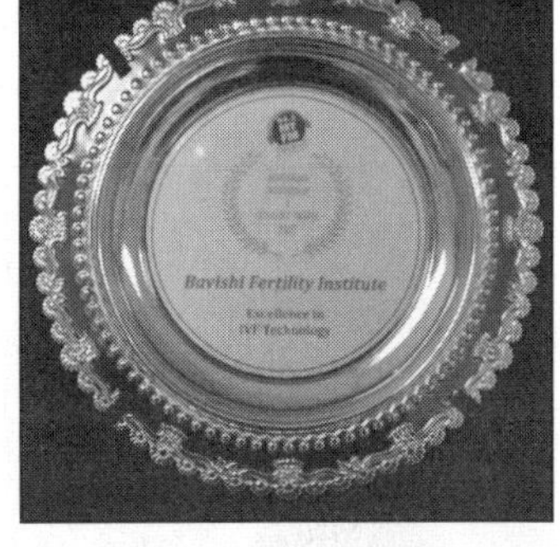

Won the 2017 'Excellence in IVF' Award from 'MY FM' Divya Bhaskar Group. Again become the fist Fertility Institute of Ahmedabad to win this prestigeous award.

Technical support: Bavishi Fertility Institute joined hands with Diamond Institute for infertility and menopause, New Jersey, USA for setting of world class IVF centre in Ahmedabad. The diamond Institute has constantly supported Bavishi

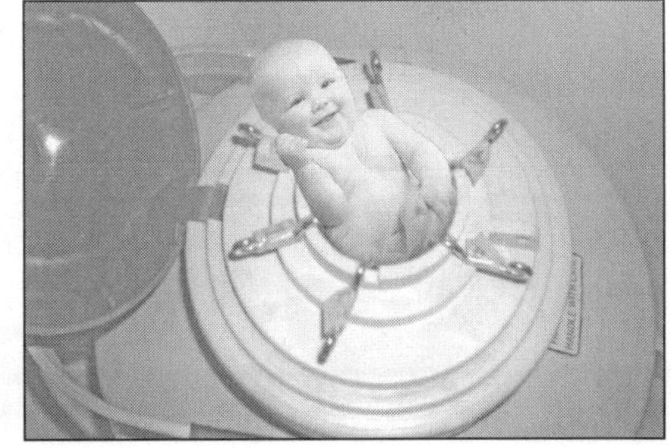

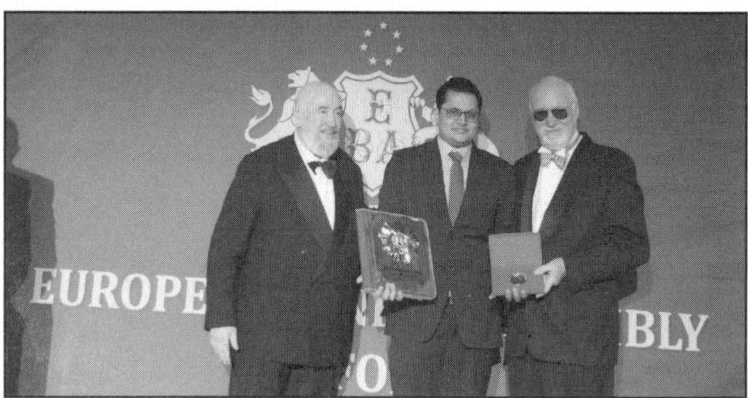

Fertility Institute on technology and training as well as scientific and public awareness programmes.

In 2008 live birth with vitrified frozen egg happened for the fist time in India at Bavishi Fertility Institute.

Bavishi Fertility Institute proudly claimed fist live birth of India with frozen egg (Vitrified oocytes). Very few live births

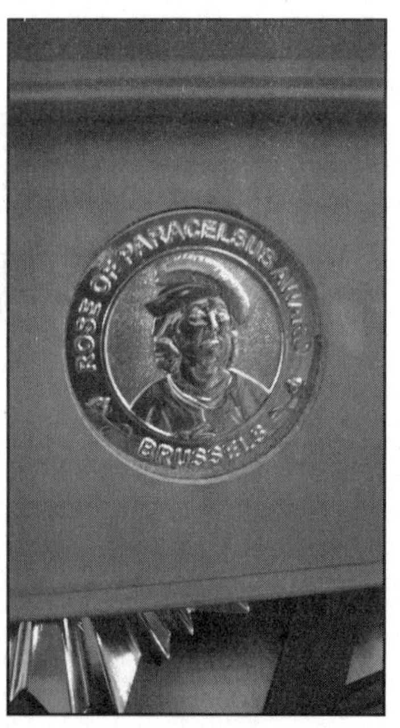

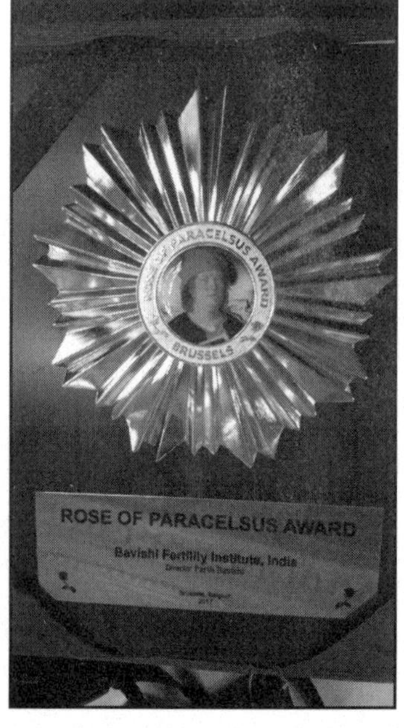

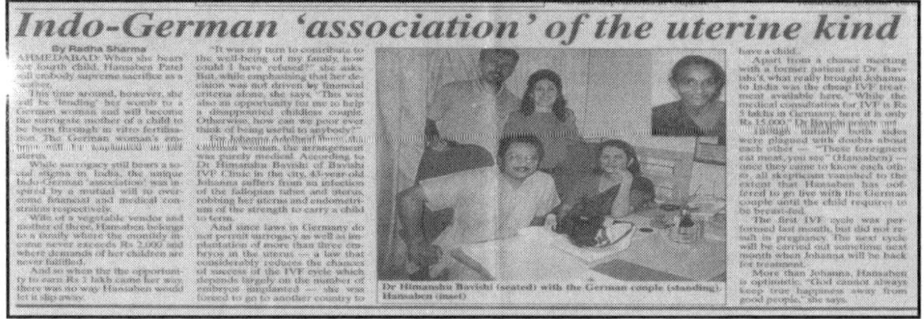

Indo-German 'association' of the uterine kind

By Radha Sharma

Dr Himanshu Bavishi (seated) with the German couple (standing). Hansaben (inset)

were recorded world over till that date. Now Bavishi Fertility Institute has successfully delivered babies through frozen egg of patients, donor and even with testicular sperm. Bavishi Fertility Institute's pioneering concept of 'Egg Bank' is now well established.

Bavishi Fertility institute received 'Socrates award - Rose of Paracelsus' from Europe Medical association on 3rd July 201 7, at Lucerne Switzerland, at an event organised by Europe Business assembly.

Pioneered in surrogacy in India

To help infertile couples who cannot become parents without the help of surrogacy, Bavishi Fertility Institute pioneered Surrogacy treatment in India. Bavishi Fertility Institute become fist institute of India to treat European couple for surrogacy in 1999. Dr. Himanshu

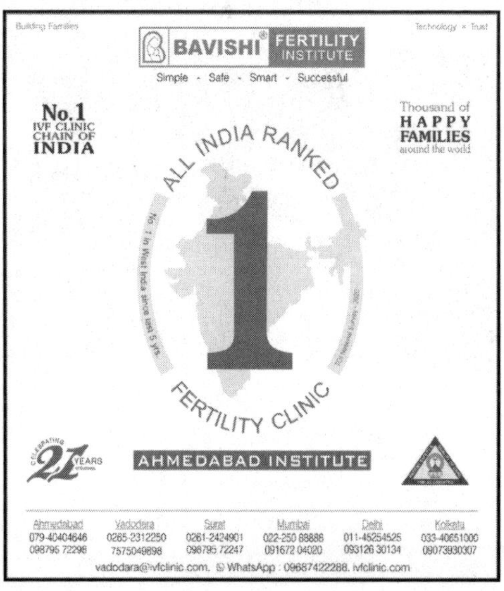

Bavishi is founder president of 'Indian Society for Third Party Assisted Reproduction'– INSTAR.

First IVF Babies Meet –2004

For fist of its kind, awareness programme, Bavishi Fertility Institute organised 'IVF Babies Meet' in 2004, to break the myths and spread awareness about the modern technology. More than 100 IVF babies conceived at Bavishi Fertility Institute, participated.

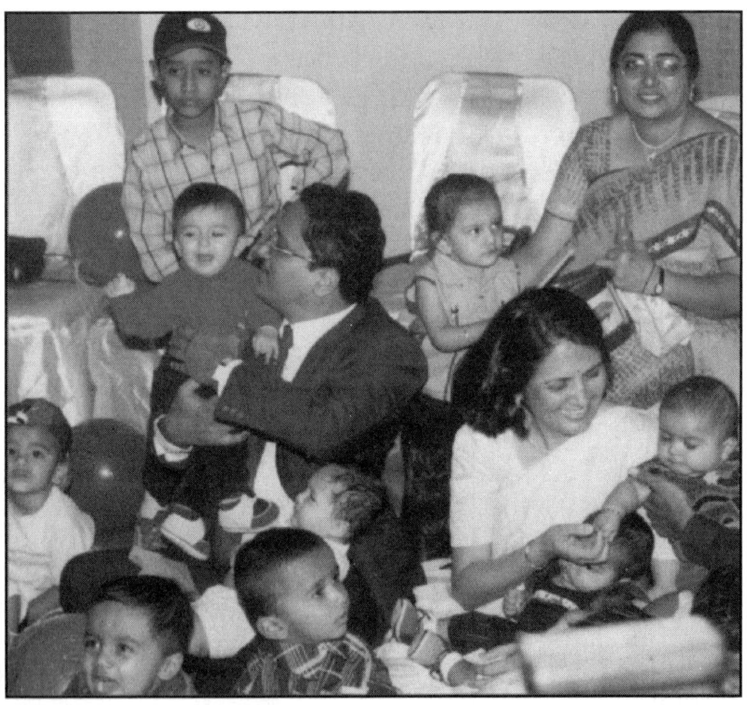

□□□